The Simplest Alkaline Diet Guide for Beginners + 45 Easy Recipes

7 Days Meal Plan to Bring Your Body Back to Balance

Sheldon Miller

Table of contents

Introduction 5
    The outlook of an Alkaline Diet 8
    The Definition of pH 10
    Understanding the harmful impacts of pH imbalance 12
    The natural way of your body to defend itself .. 14
    The amazing advantages of Alkaline Diet 16
    The Perfect Food For Alkaline Diet 17
    Foods and Habits to Refrain From 22
    Scholarly Meal Plan (7 Days) 24

Chapter 1: Breakfast Recipes 39
    Cute Pecan Pancakes #1 39
    Craving Quinoa Breakfast #2 41
    Steel Oats Of Amazement #3 43
    Flavorful Hashed Sunchokes #4 45
    Garden Variety Pancakes Of Awe #5 47
    A Tropical Sided Granola #6 49
    Summer's Ideal Salad With Mint and Lime #7 . 51
    Classical American Apple Pie #8 53
    Savage Baked Grapefruit #9 55
    Cute and Cuddly Baby Potatoes #10 57

Chapter 2: Lunch Recipes 59
    Majestic Zucchini Salad #1 59
    Coconut Milk And Glazing Stir Fried Tofu #2 ... 61

- Culturally Diverse Pumpkin Potato Patties! #3 .. 63
- Italian Leek Fry #4 65
- Almond And Celery Mix Of Delight! #5 67
- Spicy Tofu Burger (Magical) #6 69
- Special Pasta Ala Pepper and Tomato Sauce #7 71
- Southern Amazing Salad #8 73
- A Concoction of Roast Veggies #9 75
- A Thai Pad Thai #10 77

Chapter 3: Dinner Recipes 79
- Chinese Cucumber Salad Magnifico #1 79
- Mediterranean Specialty Alkaline Salad #2 81
- Emmenthal Justifiable Soup From Swiss! #3 ... 83
- Buckwheat Pasta mixed up with Bell Pepper and Broccoli #4 85
- Artichoke Sauce Ala Quinoa Pasta! #5 87
- The Mighty Indian Curry Of Lentil #6 89
- Savory Deluxe Mix Of Veggies #7 91
- Very Wild Avocado Salad #8 93
- The Mysterious Alkaline Veggies and Rice (Wilde) #9 95
- Beautifully Curried Eggplant #10 97

Chapter 4: Dessert Recipes 99
- Magnificent Coconut Ice Cream Sundae #1 99
- All Purpose Thanksgiving Pudding #2 101
- Dates For A Valentine's Day Date #3 103
- Crispy Fruit Mix #4 105

Slightly Crispy Rice Treatlets #5 107
Mystical Indian Aloo Gobi #6 109
Crazy Soy Pudding #7 111
Mouthwatering Banana Muffins #8 113
Mr. Clause's Stuffed Avocado #9 115
Gorgeous Garlic Cabbage #10 117
Chapter 5: Fantastic Smoothie Recipes 119
A Pina Colada For The Adventurers #1 119
Mango and Papaya Raspberry Smoothie #2 ... 121
Sensuous Banana Nut Bread Smoothie #3 123
Honorable Orange Potion of Health #4 125
Cherry and Chocolate Mixture #5 127
Conclusion 129

Introduction

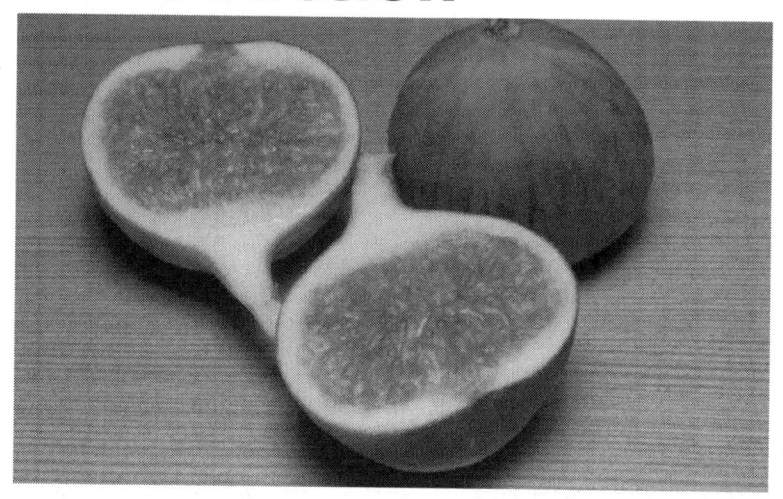

Assuming that you have already done your research on this topic, you have most likely stumbled upon different pieces of evidence that elaborate on the positive impact of alkaline diet.

The basic concept of the Alkaline Diet follows an ideology that believes that the human body turns into a very healthy metabolic machine when acidic (acid forming) foods are completely replaced with Alkaline based ones.

Without any prior knowledge, this is a concept that might seem a little bit hard to believe at first, but scientists all around the world are proving it otherwise!

In fact, the positivity of this diet has been proven to the extent that it can even fend of diseases such as Cancer.

Such results have slowly catapulted Alkaline Diet to the hearts of millions all around the world, and I am hoping that you will be the next one to learn to appreciate the magic of this diet.

And yet, Atkins diet is perhaps one of the most effective yet misunderstood diets out there right in the mainstream world!

Around the world, the alkaline diet is largely known as Alkaline-Ash diet or even Acid Ash diet as well. So, don't be confused if you see those names around! But for the sake of simplicity, throughout the book, we will be simply referring to the diet as being "Alkaline Diet"

The core aim of the diet, as mentioned earlier is to simply cut down a certain group of food that is largely considered to be "Acidic'" and provide help the dietician create a meal plan that encourages him/her to eat foods that sport an Alkaline flavor.

These mostly consist of vegetables and fruits.

I have tried my very best to make this book as much accessible and simple as possible to ensure that newcomers are able to easily digest the topic and understand the concept behind this widely misunderstood topic.

Once you have a strong grasp of the topic, you are more than welcome to explore the amazing

40+ recipes provided with the book to experiment and enjoy!

Welcome, to the amazing world of Alkaline Diet!

The outlook of an Alkaline Diet

The core principle that surrounds this diet is a simple philosophy that believes that foods that we consume can very easily alter the internal chemistry of our body, depending on whether the food is acidity or alkalinity of the food. Strictly speaking, the pH of our body changes depending on the food.

Don't just get jumbled yet though! I will be explaining the terms in details shortly.

But I will be doing a little science talk, so bear with me.

Before moving forward, you must appreciate the fact that whenever our body requires energy, it starts to burn down food. The whole process is extremely controlled and takes place in a very strict environment that is controlled by the biology of our body.

In terms of consumed foods, they also leave behind a residue which we are going to refer to as "Ash" as well.

This "Ash" actually has the potential to either be acidic, alkaline or neutral. And these residues or "Ashes" are responsible for altering the pH of our body.

The bottom line here is that if your body is exposed to a greater amount of acidic "Ash", it slowly starts to become more vulnerable to diseases as the immune system weakens.

Alternatively, when your body enjoys a high level of alkalinity in the blood stream, a sort of protective layer starts to form, which keeps tries to keep the body healthy.

For such reasons, it is highly recommended that you always try to opt for foods that are high on alkaline value.

In short, the following is a categorization of the different kinds of foods based on the state of their "Ashes"

- **Acidic:** Produces such as meat, fish, poultry, dairy, grains, eggs and even alcohol are considered to be acidic.
- **Neutral:** Foods such as sugars, fats or starches are said to be neutral
- **Alkaline:** Foods including vegetables, legume, nuts, and Fruits are said to be Alkaline.

The Definition of pH
The pH Scale

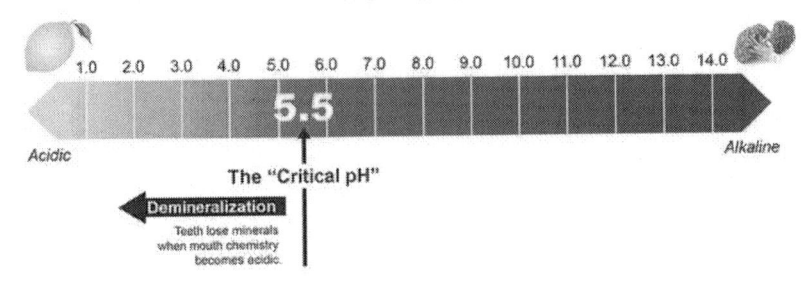

```
1.0  2.0  3.0  4.0  5.0  6.0  7.0  8.0  9.0  10.0  11.0  12.0  13.0  14.0
                    5.5
Acidic                                                            Alkaline
              The "Critical pH"
         ← Demineralization
           Teeth lose minerals
           when mouth chemistry
           becomes acidic.
```

Now that you have a firm grasp of the concept of Alkaline Diet, we are going to dive deeper into the topic.

You must now learn to appreciate the meaning of "pH".

Generally speaking, pH is a component of our blood known as the Potential of Hydrogen.

Using the value is pH; it is possible to assess if a liquid is alkaline or acidic. In the case of human beings, we measure the acidity or alkalinity of the bodily fluids and tissues.

The measurement is usually done within a scale of 0-14. The rule goes as such

- The lower the pH value, the acidic a solution is
- The higher the value goes, the more alkaline the solution is
- 7 is considered to be the neutral point on the scale

The pH level of our body normally stays at 7.4 which is considered to be a safe point. However, it has been deduced that if the pH level goes to the point of being slightly alkaline, the overall health condition seems to improve a lot.

It should be noted though that the pH level of the body varies from one region to the next. For example, the stomach is generally regarded as naturally being the most acidic part of the body.

If the natural level of pH gets altered by even a slight amount, the body of human beings, as well as many other organisms, starts to react negatively.

A good example would be the recent increase of Carbon Di-Oxide disposition which led to a large a slight decrease in the ocean's pH, where it went to 8.1 from 8.2

And 0.1 change in pH, various aquatic organism and life forms have started to suffer.

This pH level is not only essential for plant growth, but also the minerals in our food.

But every single organism has some kind of means of defending the body from such changes. In case of human beings, various minerals contribute by acting as a "buffer" to normalize the pH level of our body should it become more acidic!

Understanding the harmful impacts of pH imbalance

By now, you should have a clear idea of the importance of maintaining a balanced body pH! This section is to give you an idea of the fatal consequences of pH changes.

For example, if the pH level of your body becomes too alkaline, then Alkalosis will take place. Under such conditions, you will start to experience loss of electrolytes, lower oxygen levels, liver disease, etc.

Symptoms of Alkalosis includes

- Confusion
- Lightheadedness
- Twitching
- Sudden muscle spasm
- Seizure
- Respiratory problems
- Tingling in facial extremities

Consequently, if your body condition starts to become too acidic, then your body will start to enter a state called "Acidosis". Some risk of Acidosis include

Symptoms of Acidosis

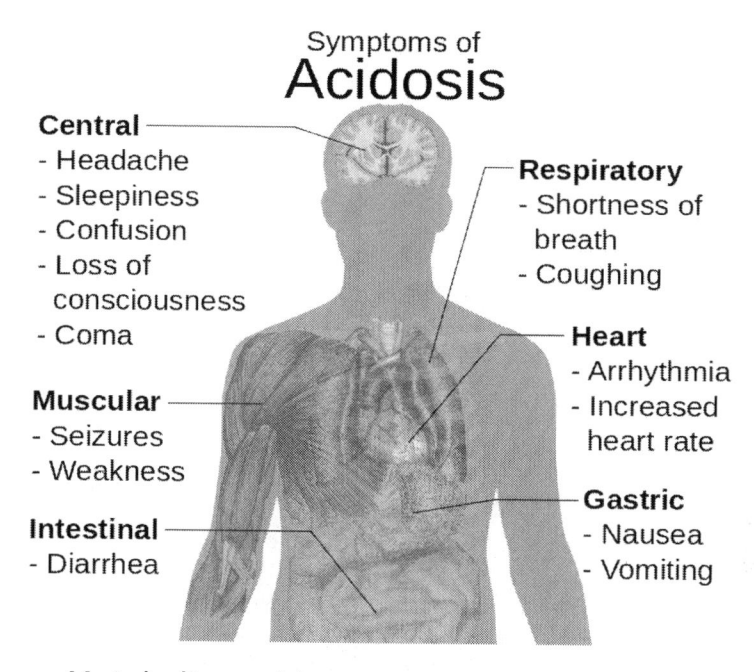

Central
- Headache
- Sleepiness
- Confusion
- Loss of consciousness
- Coma

Muscular
- Seizures
- Weakness

Intestinal
- Diarrhea

Respiratory
- Shortness of breath
- Coughing

Heart
- Arrhythmia
- Increased heart rate

Gastric
- Nausea
- Vomiting

- Metabolic problems
- Respiratory problems
- Lactic imbalance
- Renal complications
- Increased risk of cardiovascular diseases
- Diabetes
- Insulin Resistance
- Kidney Damage
- Confusion
- Fatigue
- Breathlessness
- Lethargy

In fact, Acidosis may very well be induced by an improper diet containing a lot of animal products with a few fruits and vegetables.

The natural way of your body to defend itself

Our body has been fully equipped with the means to tackle itself from such changes to keep it protected, should the pH level change.

Kidneys are the main line of defense when it comes to dealing with Acidosis.

Whenever the acid level increases, the Kidney starts to send the excess acid to our bladder, which is later on excreted through urination.

The kidney also helps to maintain the levels of bicarbonate that greatly helps the body to tackle the acidic effects as well.

In worst case scenarios, if the kidneys start to fail or get compromised and fail to control the acid levels, then the body will start to experience serious complications.

Early on, these complications won't be serious; however, they will increase with time.

You should know though that the filtration process of the kidney isn't the only part of your body that helps to maintain the pH level.

In fact, the lungs play a great role too.

Carbon Di Oxide is the by-product of cellular metabolism, but the problem occurs if it starts to get mixed with the blood as it causes it to become acidic.

The lungs help to get rid of the CO2 from our body, helping to maintain a balance of acid-base in our body.

The amazing advantages of Alkaline Diet

- It helps to protect your muscle density and bone mass of body
- It greatly lowers down the risk of facing hypertension and stroke
- Greatly helps to lower down inflammation and Chronic pain
- Helps to boost the absorption of Vitamin and minimizes Magnesium Deficiency
- It greatly helps to improve the immunity of the body and protects it from developing cancer
- It helps to lose weight
- An Alkaline diet will greatly increase the available energy of the body and keeps it energized all throughout the day
- It improves the health of gum and teeth
- It slows down the natural process of aging and keeps you looking younger and fresher for long
- It enhances your sexual power and increase the sexual drive

The Perfect Food For Alkaline Diet

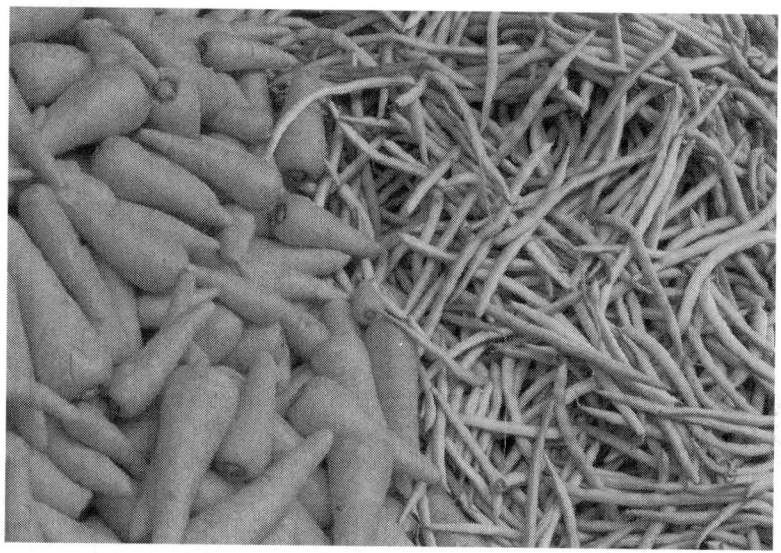

Generally speaking, your diet should comprise of fruits and vegetables alongside some grain. The following is a list that should give you an idea of the ingredients that are a "Go-Go" for your alkaline diet!

Alkaline Fruits

- Apple
- Apricot
- Avocado
- Banana
- Berries
- Blackberries
- Cantaloupe
- Cherry
- Coconut

- Currant
- Dried Date
- Dried Fig
- Grape
- Grapefruit
- Honeydew Lemon
- Lemon
- Lime
- Muskmelon
- Nectarine
- Orange
- Peach
- Pear
- Pineapple
- Raisins
- Raspberry
- Rhubarb
- Strawberry
- Tomato
- Tropical Fruits
- Watermelon
- Tangerine

Alkaline Proteins

- Almond
- Chestnut
- Millet
- Fermented Tempeh
- Fermented Tofu
- Whey Protein Powder

Alkaline Seasoning and/or Spices

- Chili Pepper
- Cinnamon
- Curry
- Ginger
- All Kinds Of Herbs
- Miso
- Mustard
- Sea Salt
- Tamari

Alkaline Sweeteners

- Stevia

Alkaline Veggies

- Alfalfa
- Barley Grass
- Beet Greens
- Beets
- Broccoli
- Cabbage
- Carrot
- Cauliflower
- Celery
- Chard Greens
- Chlorella
- Collard Greens
- Cucumber
- Daikon
- Dandelion
- Dandelion Root
- Dulce
- Edible Flowers

- Eggplant
- Garlic
- Green Beans
- Green Peas
- Kale
- Kombu
- Lettuce
- Mustard Greens
- Maitake
- Mushrooms
- Mustard Greens
- Nori
- Onions
- Parsnips
- Pea
- Pepper
- Radish
- Pumpkin
- Reishi
- Sea Vegetables
- Shiitake
- Spinach
- Sprouts
- Sweet Potatoes
- Tomato
- Wakame
- Watercress
- Wheat Grass
- Wild Greens

Some additional produces

- Apple Cider Vinegar

- Bee Pollen
- Fresh Fruit juice
- Lecithin Granules
- Backstrap Molasses
- Probiotic Cultures
- Soured Dairy Products
- Vegetable Juices
- Alkaline Antioxidant Water
- Mineral Water

Foods and Habits to Refrain From

Let me elaborate on the foods first. So, in general, you should try to avoid

- Processed foods that are high in sodium as they greatly cause the blood vessels of becoming constricted and results in acidity
- Conventional meats or Cold Cut meats
- Processed Cereals such like Chocos or Corn Flakes
- Eggs
- Lentils
- Alcohol and Caffeinated Beverages
- Produces made of grain, regardless of being "Whole' grain or not.
- Products that are extremely rich in Calcium can lead to severe cases of Osteoporosis! And this is because they are potent in creating an extremely acidic condition inside the body! And if your blood stream starts to become more acidic, they will slowly start to decay the calcium from the bones in order to balance out the pH level. Leafy vegetables are therefore the way to go when it comes to tackling osteoporosis.
- Walnuts and Peanuts
- Rice, Pasta or any other package products made of "Grain"

Aside from the restricted foods, you should also try to keep yourself away from certain habits that are also considered to thrust your body into a more Alkaline condition.

- Refrain yourself from usage of drugs or alcohol
- Prevent yourself from consuming large quantities of caffeine
- Prevent yourself from using large number of antibiotics
- Try to avoid artificial sweeteners
- Try to keep yourself free from chronic stress
- Try to maintain a good fiber intake
- Avoiding exercise
- Going for excess animal meat mostly from inorganic sources
- Ingestion of hormones through artificial means such as medicines or beauty products
- Exposing our body to radiation from cleaners, computers, microwaves, cell phones
- Using preservatives of any form of food coloring
- Getting exposed to herbicides or pesticides
- Extreme cases of pollution
- Eating refined or "processed" foods
- Breathing shallowly

Scholarly Meal Plan (7 Days)

The following is sample Alkaline meal plan that you can follow to ensure that your body remains healthy!

Keep in mind that you may mix and match the plan as required.

Most new comers tend to follow the 80/20 plan where an individual is required to make a diet that is comprised of 80% alkaline foods and 20% acidic foods.

So the choice lies completely on you!

Day 1

Breakfast	**Cute Pecan Pancakes** - Calories: 250 - Fats: 19g - Carbs:8g - Fiber:3g
Smoothie	**A Pina Colada For The Adventures** - Calories: 175 - Fats: 3.2g - Carbs: 38g - Fiber: 3.8g
Lunch	**Special Pasta Ala Pepper and Tomato Sauce** - Calories: 591 - Fats: 22g - Carbs: 73g - Fiber: 5g

Dinner	**Mediterranean Specialty Alkaline Salad** - Calories: 204 - Fats: 16g - Carbs: 10g - Fiber: 1g
Desert	**Slightly Crispy Rice Treatles** - Calories: 104 - Fats: 4.6g - Carbs: 15g - Fiber: 4.6g

Day 2

Breakfast	**Steel Oats Of Amazement** - Calories: 231 - Fats: 5g - Carbs: 38g - Fiber: 6g
Snack	**Mango and Papaya Raspberry Smoothie** - Calories: 175 - Fats: 3.2g - Carbs: 38g - Fiber: 3.8g
Lunch	**Almond And Celery Mix Of Delight** - Calories: 221 - Fats: 15g - Carbs: 23g - Fiber: 3g

Dinner	**Buckwheat Pasta Mixed Up With Bell Pepper and Broccoli** - Calories: 583 - Fats: 26g - Carbs:61g - Fiber: 4g
Desert	**Crispy Fruit Mix** - Calories: 240 - Fats: 16g - Carbs: 20g - Fiber: 5.8g

Day 3

Breakfast	**Garden Variety Pancake Of Awe** - Calories: 254 - Fats: 12g - Carbs: 33g - Fiber: 7g
Smoothie	**Sensuous Banana Nut Bread Smoothie** - Calories: 254 - Fats: 12g - Carbs: 33g - Fiber: 7.2g
Lunch	**Culturally Diverse Pumpkin Potato Patties** - Calories: 375 - Fats: 16g - Carbs: 46g - Fiber: 7g

Dinner	**The Mighty Indian Curry Of Lentil** - Calories: 421 - Fats: 6g - Carbs: 79g - Fiber: 59g
Desert	**Dates For A Valentine Day Date** - Calories: 178 - Fats: 8g - Carbs: 27g - Fiber: 4.3g

Day 4

Breakfast	**Classical American Apple Pie** - Calories: 109 - Fats: 0.1g - Carbs: 28g - Fiber: 4g
Smoothie	**Honorable Orange Potion Of Health** - Calories: 184 - Fats: 0.3g - Carbs: 44g - Fiber: 3.8g
Lunch	**Majestic Zucchini Salad** - Calories: 109 - Fats: 0.1g - Carbs: 28g - Fiber: 4g

Dinner	**Magnificent Ice Cream Sundae** - Calories: 306 - Fats: 22g - Carbs: 30g - Fiber: 2.6g
Desert	**The Indian Lassi With Strawberry** - Calories: 180 - Fat: 9g - Carbohydrates: 23g - Protein: 4g - Dietary Fiber: 3g

Day 5

Breakfast	**Steel Oats Of Amazement** - Calories: 231 - Fats: 5g - Carbs: 38g - Fiber: 6g
Snack	**Mango and Papaya Raspberry Smoothie** - Calories: 175 - Fats: 3.2g - Carbs: 38g - Fiber: 3.8g
Lunch	**Almond And Celery Mix Of Delight** - Calories: 221 - Fats: 15g - Carbs: 23g - Fiber: 3g

Dinner	**Buckwheat Pasta Mixed Up With Bell Pepper and Broccoli** - Calories: 583 - Fats: 26g - Carbs: 61g - Fiber: 4g
Desert	**Crispy Fruit Mix** - Calories: 240 - Fats: 16g - Carbs: 20g - Fiber: 5.8g

Day 6

Breakfast	**Garden Variety Pancake Of Awe** - Calories: 254 - Fats: 12g - Carbs: 33g - Fiber: 7g
Smoothie	**Sensuous Banana Nut Bread Smoothie** - Calories: 254 - Fats: 12g - Carbs: 33g - Fiber: 7.2g
Lunch	**Culturally Diverse Pumpkin Potato Patties** - Calories: 375 - Fats: 16g - Carbs: 46g - Fiber: 7g

Dinner	**The Mighty Indian Curry Of Lentil** - Calories: 421 - Fats: 6g - Carbs: 79g - Fiber: 59g
Desert	**Dates For A Valentine Day Date** - Calories: 178 - Fats: 8g - Carbs: 27g - Fiber: 4.3g

Day 7

Breakfast	**Classical American Apple Pie** - Calories: 109 - Fats: 0.1g - Carbs: 28g - Fiber: 4g
Smoothie	**Honorable Orange Potion Of Health** - Calories: 184 - Fats: 0.3g - Carbs: 44g - Fiber: 3.8g
Lunch	**Majestic Zucchini Salad** - Calories: 109 - Fats: 0.1g - Carbs: 28g - Fiber: 4g

Dinner	**Magnificent Ice Cream Sundae** - Calories: 306 - Fats: 22g - Carbs: 30g - Fiber: 2.6g
Desert	**The Indian Lassi With Strawberry** - Calories: 180 - Fat: 9g - Carbohydrates: 23g - Protein: 4g - Dietary Fiber: 3g

Chapter 1: Breakfast Recipes

Cute Pecan Pancakes #1

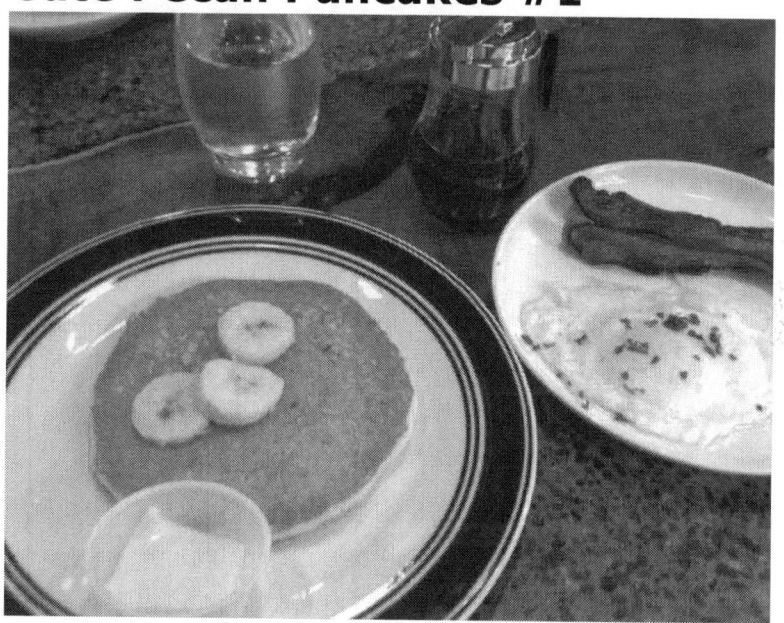

Serving: 5

Prep Time: 5 minutes

Cook Time: 30

Ingredients

- Olive oil cooking spray as needed
- ¾ cup of Atkins Cuisine All Purpose Baking Mix
- 1 tablespoon of Granular Sugar Substitute
- ½ a teaspoon of baking powder
- ¼ teaspoon of salt

- 2 large sized eggs
- ¾ cup of unsweetened soy milk
- 2 tablespoon of melted unsalted butter
- 1 teaspoon of pure vanilla extract
- ½ a teaspoon of ground cinnamon
- ¼ teaspoon of ground nutmeg
- ¼ cup of chopped toasted pecans

Cooking Directions

1. Take a large sized bowl and add baking mix, baking powder, sugar substitute, salt and mix well
2. Take another bowl and whisk eggs, butter, soy milk and vanilla
3. Pour the egg mixture into the dry mixture bowl
4. Stir well
5. Add cinnamon, pecans, and nutmegs
6. Stir for another 5 minutes
7. Take 12-inch skillet and spray it with cooking spray
8. Place it over medium high heat
9. Scoop 1 heaping tablespoon of batter into the pan and use the back of your spoon to make a 4-inch circle
10. Repeat the process 3 times and cook for 3 minutes until bubbles form at the edges and the bottoms are golden brown
11. Flip it up and cook for another 2 minutes
12. Repeat the process with the rest of the batter
13. Serve with sugar-free pancake syrup or syrup

Nutrition Values

- Calories: 250
- Fats: 19g
- Carbs: 8g
- Fiber: 3g

Craving Quinoa Breakfast #2

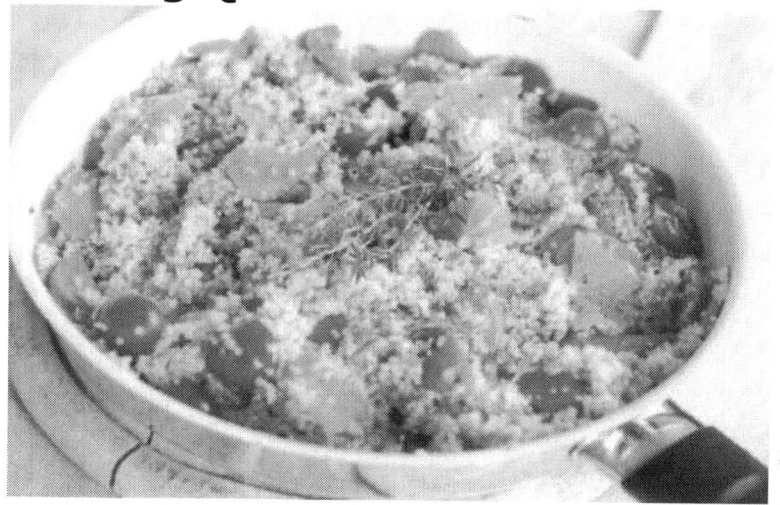

Serving: 4

Prep Time: 5 minutes

Cook Time: 15

Ingredients

- 1 cup of quinoa
- 2 cups of water
- 1 piece of 2 inches sized cinnamon stick
- 2-3 tablespoon of maple syrup

For added flavor

- ½ cup of blueberries, raspberries or strawberries
- 2 tablespoon of raisins
- 1 teaspoon of lime
- ¼ teaspoon of freshly grated nutmeg
- 3 tablespoon of whipped coconut cream
- 2 tablespoon of chopped cashew nuts
- Yogurt if desired

Cooking Directions

1. Take a metal strainer and pass your grain through them to strain them well
2. Rinse the grains under cold water thoroughly
3. Take a medium sized saucepan and pour water
4. Add the strained grains and bring the whole mixture to a boil
5. Add cinnamon sticks and cover the saucepan
6. Lower down the heat and let the mixture simmer for 15 minutes to allow the grain to absorb the liquid
7. Remove the heat and fluff up the mixture using a fork
8. Add maple syrup if you want additional flavor
9. Also, if you are looking to make things a bit more interesting, just add any of the ingredients mentioned above

Nutrition Values

- Calories: 223
- Fats: 5g
- Carbs: 37g
- Fiber: 8g

Steel Oats Of Amazement #3

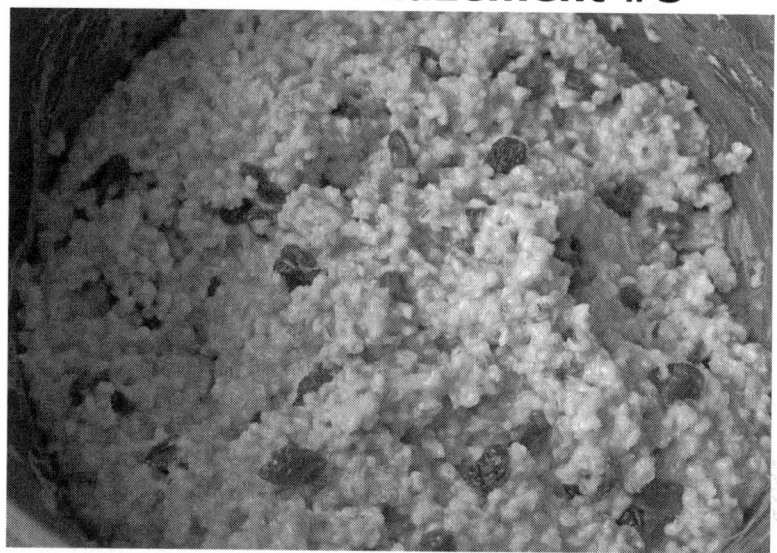

Serving: 4

Prep Time: 5 minutes

Cook Time: 15

Ingredients

- 3 and a ¾ cup of water
- 1 and a ¼ cup of steel-cut oats
- ¼ teaspoon of salt

For added flavor

- 1 teaspoon of cinnamon
- ½ a teaspoon of nutmeg
- ½ teaspoon of lemon pepper
- 1 teaspoon of Garam masala
- Mixed berries
- Diced mangos
- Sliced bananas

- Dried Fruits
- Nuts

For creaminess

- 1 tablespoon of coconut milk

Cooking Directions

1. Take a medium sized sauce pan and bring it over high heat
2. Add water and allow the water to heat up
3. Add the steel cut oats with some salt and lower down the heat to medium-low
4. Let the mixture simmer for about 25 minutes, making sure to keep stirring it from all the way
5. Add coconut milk or almond butter for some extra flavor
6. Once done, serve with some berries or nuts
7. Enjoy!

Nutrition Values

- Calories: 231
- Fats: 5g
- Carbs: 38g
- Fiber: 6g

Flavorful Hashed Sunchokes #4

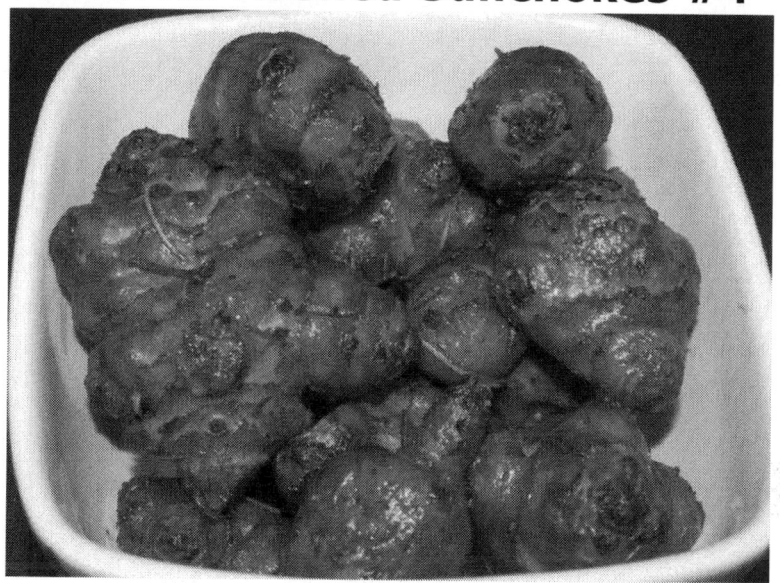

Serving: 4

Prep Time: 10 minutes

Cook Time: 6 minutes

Ingredients

- 3-4 pieces of finely sliced up and well blanched Sunchokes
- 5-6 pieces of thinly sliced up Brussels sprouts
- Seas salt as needed
- Ground pepper as needed
- Drizzle of truffle oil or extra virgin olive oil with rosemary infused in
- Finely slice up spring onion for garnish

Cooking Directions

1. Take a bowl and add cold water

2. Take the Sunchokes and slice them up
3. Dip the slices into cold water and let the rest
4. Rinse them thoroughly for about 3 times and pat them dry using a kitchen towel very carefully
5. Take a pan and place it over medium heat
6. Pour ghee/oil
7. Add the sliced up Brussels sprouts and the drained Sunchokes
8. Saute for about 4 minutes until fully cooked
9. Once done, take them out and serve!
10. As an alternative option, you are allowed to chop up your chokes and add them to a highly heated girdle
11. Cook them well to prepare your hash
12. And you are ready!

Nutrition Values

- Calories: 279
- Fats: 18g
- Carbs: 28g
- Fiber: 3g

Garden Variety Pancakes Of Awe #5

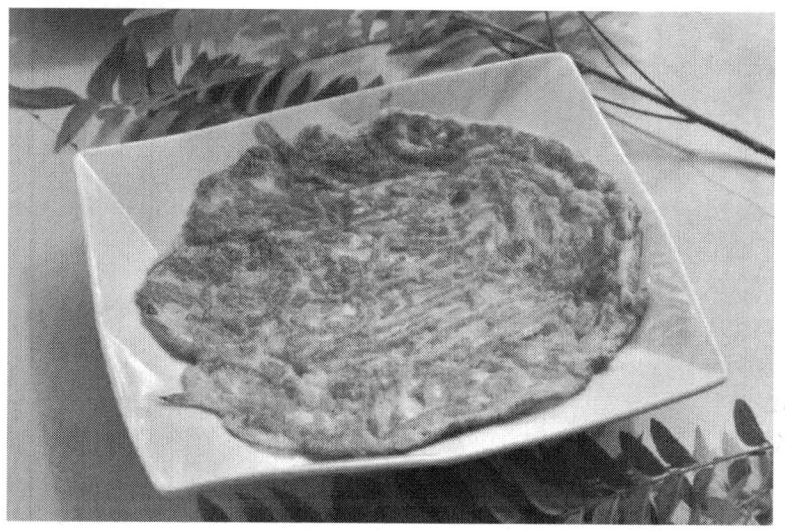

Serving: 2

Prep Time: 5 minutes

Cook Time: 5 minutes

Ingredients

- 1 medium sized roughly chopped zucchini
- 1 peeled and roughly chopped carrot
- 1 roughly chopped yellow squash
- ½ of a grated small onion
- 4 scallions
- ¼ cup of almond flour
- 1 teaspoon of sea salt
- ½ a teaspoon of garlic powder
- ¼ cup of filtered water
- Cooking spray for greasing pan

Cooking Directions

1. Take your food processor and add carrot, zucchini, yellow squash, almond flour, scallions, salt and garlic powder
2. Pulse them until they are fully blended
3. Add water to ensure that the mixture is just moist yet fairly thick
4. Take a large sized skillet and grease it up, place it over medium high heat
5. Once oil is hot, add the mixture using an ice cream scoop and brown them for about 5 minutes (giving 2 and a half minute for each side)
6. Use a fork to ensure that the batter is spread evenly

Nutrition Values

- Calories: 254
- Fats: 12g
- Carbs: 33g
- Fiber: 7g

A Tropical Sided Granola #6

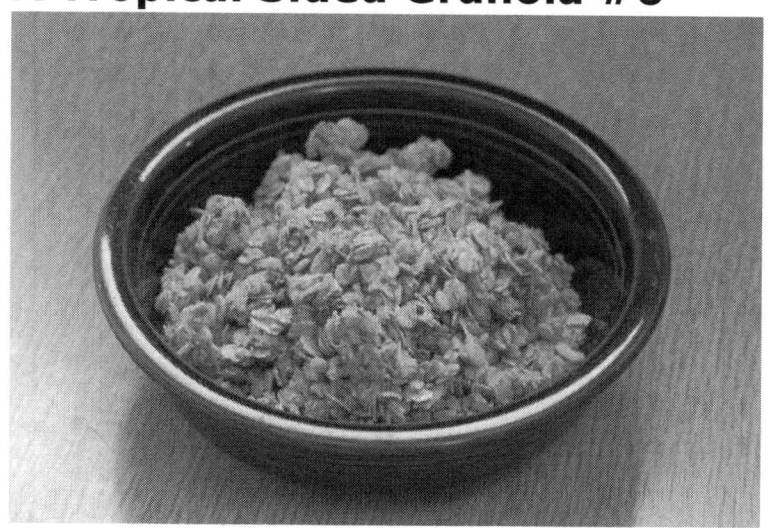

Serving: 4

Prep Time: 2 minutes

Cook Time: 15 minutes

Ingredients

- 1 cup of unsweetened coconut flaked
- 1 cup of slivered almonds
- ½ a cup of flax seed
- ½ a cup of raisins
- ½ a teaspoon of cinnamon
- ¼ teaspoon of ginger
- ¼ teaspoon of nutmeg
- ¼ teaspoon of sea salt
- 1 vanilla bean (split lengthwise, and seeds scraped out)
- ¼ cup of coconut oil
- ½ a cup of unsweetened dried pineapple tidbits

Cooking Directions

1. Preheat your oven to a temperature of 350 degrees Fahrenheit
2. Take a medium sized bowl and add coconut, flaxseed, coconut, cinnamon, raisins, ginger, salt, nutmeg, vanilla bean seeds and coconut oil
3. Toss everything until they are finely mixed
4. Spread the mix carefully and evenly on a baking sheet and transfer it to your pre-heated oven
5. Bake for 15 minutes making sure to keep stirring it from time to time
6. Remove it from the oven and let it cool
7. Once done, stir in your pineapple tidbits and serve!

Nutrition Values

- Calories: 293
- Fats: 0.3g
- Carbs: 44g
- Fiber: 3.8g

Summer's Ideal Salad With Mint and Lime #7

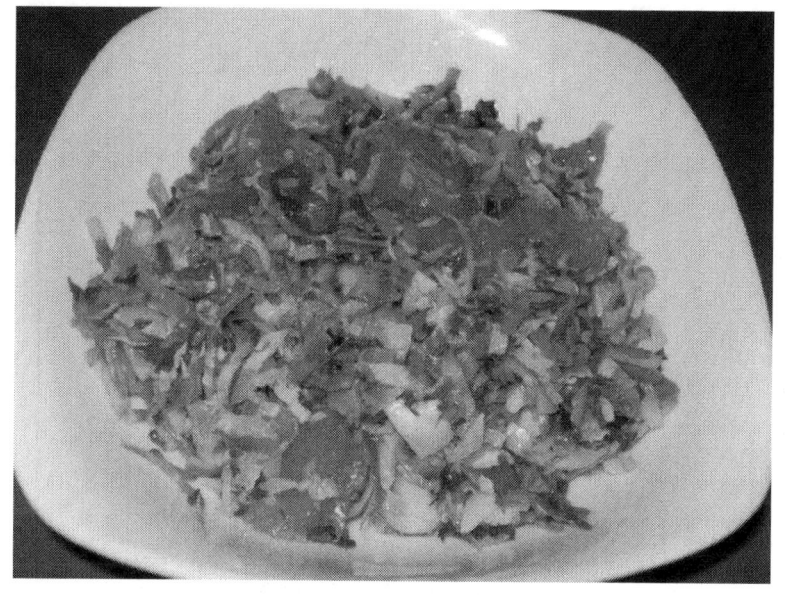

Serving: 4

Prep Time: 10 minutes

Cook Time: 0 minutes

Ingredients

- ¼ cup of grapes
- ¼ cup of peeled and diced apple
- ¼ cup of bite sized watermelon pieces
- ¼ cup of bite sized honeydew melon pieces
- ¼ cup of bite sized cantaloupe pieces
- ¼ cup of tangerine slices
- ¼ cup of peeled and diced peaches
- ¼ cup of strawberries
- 2 tablespoon of chopped fresh mint
- 2 tablespoon of freshly squeezed lemon juice

Cooking Directions

1. Take a medium sized bowl and add grapes, watermelon, apple, honeydew, tangerine, strawberries, peaches, and cantaloupe
2. Add lemon juice and mint
3. Mix everything well and cover it up
4. Let it chill overnight and serve!

Nutrition Values

- Calories: 32
- Fats: 0.2g
- Carbs:8g
- Fiber: 0.9g

Classical American Apple Pie #8

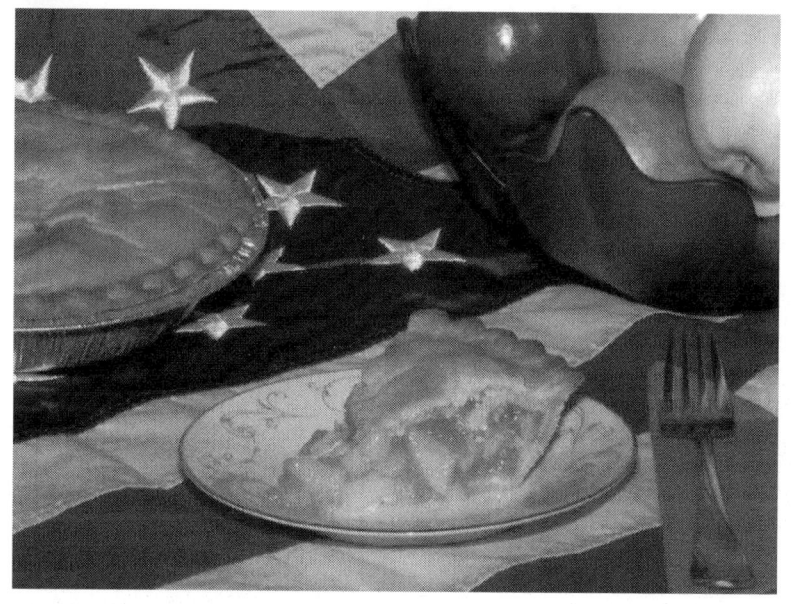

Serving: 4

Prep Time: 10 minutes

Cook Time: 10 minutes

Ingredients

- 4 golden delicious apples (cored and sliced)
- ½ a cup of freshly squeezed orange juice
- 1 vanilla bean split lengthwise
- ¼ teaspoon of cinnamon
- Unsweetened coconut milk

Cooking Directions

1. Take a large sized bowl and add apples alongside orange juice, cinnamon, and vanilla bean seeds

2. Take a medium sized skillet and place it over medium heat
3. Add fruit mixture and cook for 10 minutes until the apples are fully caramelized
4. Divide the mix amongst four serving dish
5. Serve warm with a topping of coconut milk

<u>Nutrition Values</u>

- Calories: 109
- Fats: 0.1g
- Carbs:28g
- Fiber: 4g

Savage Baked Grapefruit #9

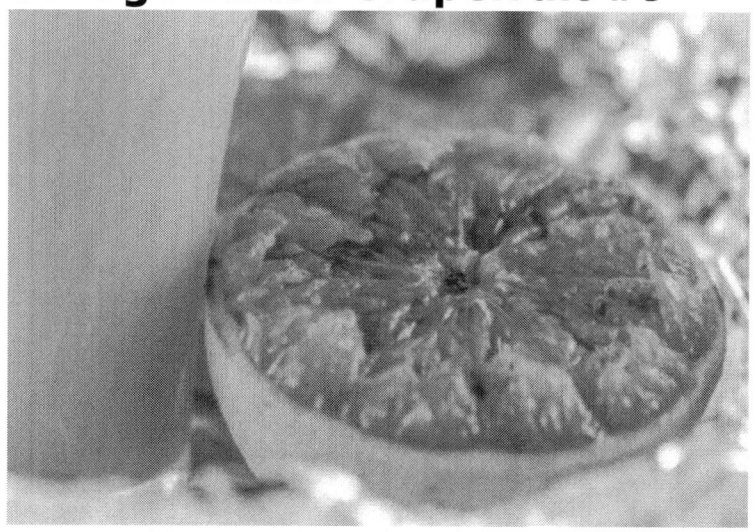

Serving: 1

Prep Time: 15 minutes

Cook Time: 15 minutes

Ingredients

- 1 halved grapefruit
- 2 tablespoon of unsweetened grated coconut

Cooking Directions

1. Preheat your oven to a temperature of 350 degrees Fahrenheit
2. Take a baking pan and line it up with foil
3. Add the grapefruit halves and top each of them with 1 tablespoon of coconut
4. Add the pan to your pre-heated oven and bake for 15 minutes
5. Wait until the coconuts are nicely browned
6. Serve and enjoy!

Nutrition Values

- Calories: 86
- Fats: 0.7g
- Carbs: 11g
- Fiber: 2.3g

Cute and Cuddly Baby Potatoes #10

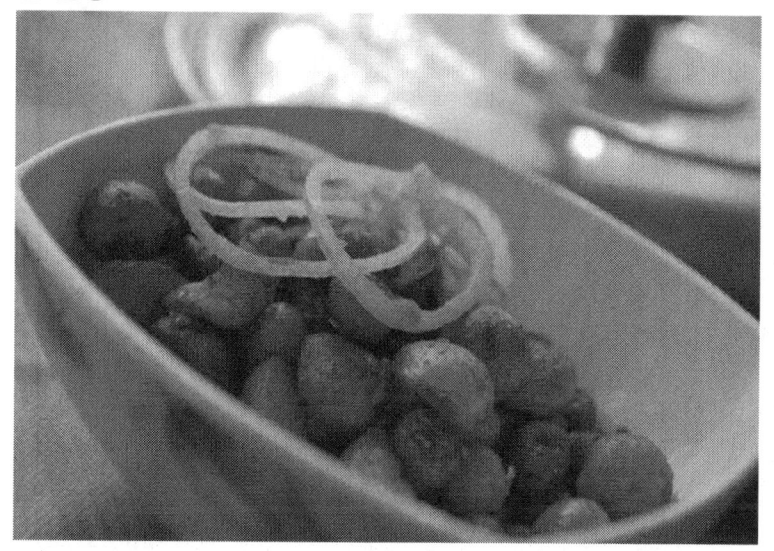

Serving: 2

Prep Time: 5 minutes

Cook Time: 20 minutes

Ingredients

- 4 medium sized baby white potatoes
- 2 ounce of vegetable broth
- ½ of a chopped sweet white onion
- 1 seeded and diced red bell pepper
- ½ a cup of sliced mushrooms
- 1 teaspoon of sea salt
- 1 teaspoon of garlic powder

Cooking Directions

1. Take a medium sized microwave-safe bowl and microwave your potatoes for about 4 minutes to allow them to be tender
2. Take a large sized non-skillet and place it over medium heat
3. Add onion, broth, and red bell pepper and Saute for 5 minutes
4. Cut the potatoes into quarter
5. Add the quartered potatoes to the skillet alongside mushrooms, garlic powder, and salt
6. Stir well
7. Cook for 10 minutes until the potatoes are crisp
8. Serve!

Nutrition Values

- Calories: 337
- Fats: 0.8g
- Carbs: 74g
- Fiber: 12g

Chapter 2: Lunch Recipes

Majestic Zucchini Salad #1

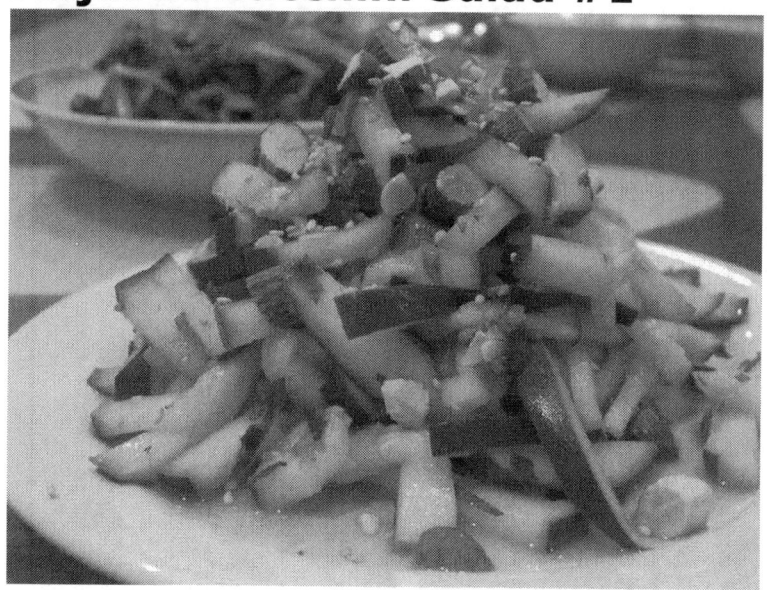

Serving: 2

Prep Time: 10 minutes

Cook Time: 0 minutes

Ingredients

- 1 piece of fresh Zucchini
- 1 piece of red bell pepper
- 2 pieces of tomatoes
- 1 piece of onion
- 1 piece clove of garlic
- ½ of a fresh lemon

- 2 tablespoon of cold pressed extra virgin olive oil
- Just a pinch of salt
- Just a pinch of pepper
- 1 teaspoon of fresh herbs

Cooking Directions

1. Wash your Zucchini under cold water well and cut up the upper portion alongside the bottom part of your zucchini
2. Cut up the zucchini lengthwise and slice up the halves crosswise
3. Take your tomatoes and wash them well, dice them up
4. Wash the bell peppers as well and cut them in half. Cut up the half into slices
5. Cut the onions into rings
6. Add veggies to a medium sized salad bowl
7. Take another bowl and add lemon juice, minced up garlic, olive oil, fresh herbs, salt and pepper
8. Pour the mixture over your salad as dressing
9. Toss and enjoy!

Nutrition Values

- Calories: 35
- Fats: 7g
- Carbs: 7g
- Fiber: 1g

Coconut Milk And Glazing Stir Fried Tofu #2

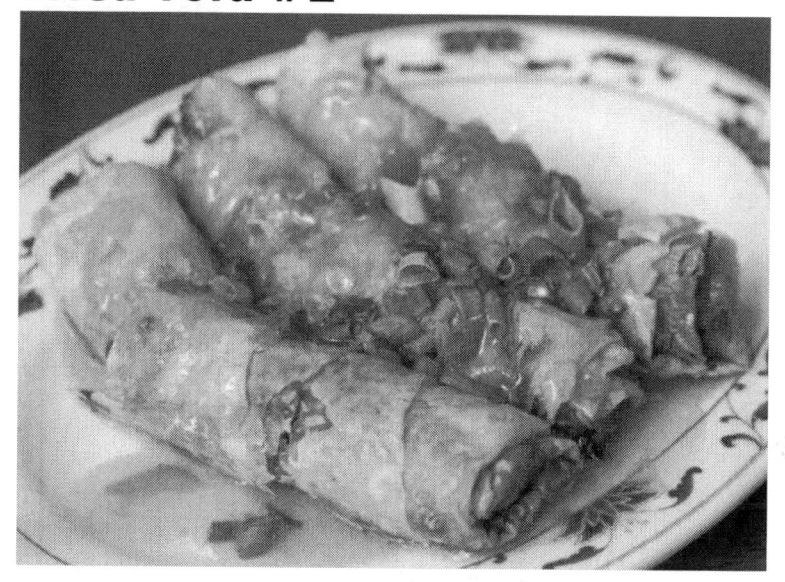

Serving: 4

Prep Time: 10 minutes

Cook Time: 5 minutes

Ingredients

- 1 pound of firm tofu
- 3 medium sized Zucchinis
- 3 pieces of tomatoes
- 1 piece of red bell pepper
- 1 piece of green bell pepper
- ½ a pound of green beans
- 1 to 1 and a ½ cup of fresh coconut milk
- 2 tablespoon of cold pressed extra virgin olive oil
- Sea salt as needed
- Pepper as needed

- ½ a tablespoon of curry powder
- ¼ tablespoon of ginger
- Fresh assorted selection of Herbs

Cooking Directions

1. Dice your tofu
2. Chop up your zucchinis
3. Chop up the bell peppers, tomatoes, beans into small portions
4. Take a pan and place it over medium heat, add oil and heat it up
5. Add tofu and fry them for about 2-3 minutes
6. Add pepper bell, beans, zucchini and stir fry for 2-3 minutes
7. Add tomatoes and coconut milk and stir well and cook for a while
8. Season with some ginger, salt, pepper, curry powder, and herbs
9. Serve with some wild rice or soba noodles
10. Have fun!

Nutrition Values

- Calories: 210
- Fats: 17g
- Carbs: 8g
- Fiber: 3g

Culturally Diverse Pumpkin Potato Patties! #3

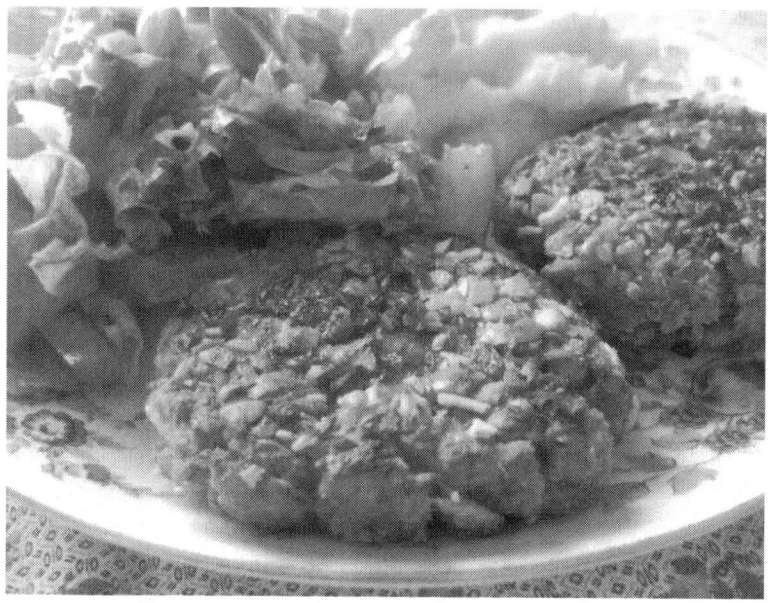

Serving: 2

Prep Time: 10 minutes

Cook Time: 5 minutes

Ingredients

- 1 pound of 450g pumpkin
- 1 pound of 450g potatoes
- 2.5 ounce of soy 75g soy flour
- 4 tablespoon of water
- 3 tablespoon of chopped up parsley
- Sea salt as needed
- Organic salt as needed
- Just a pinch of pepper
- Cold Pressed Extra virgin olive oil

Cooking Directions

1. Peel the skin of your pumpkin and potatoes
2. Take a grater and grate both of them into chunky pieces
3. Take a bowl and add 2 tablespoons of soy flour and 4 tablespoons of water
4. Take another bowl and add your grated potatoes and pumpkin alongside soy flour
5. Add flour to the mix and mix them well
6. Season with a bit of salt, parsley, and pepper
7. Take a pan and place it over medium heat. Add oil and heat it up
8. Prepare patties from the mixture and fry them in hot oil for about 2-3 minutes until they are brown
9. Serve!

Nutrition Values

- Calories: 375
- Fats: 16g
- Carbs: 46g
- Fiber: 7g

Italian Leek Fry #4

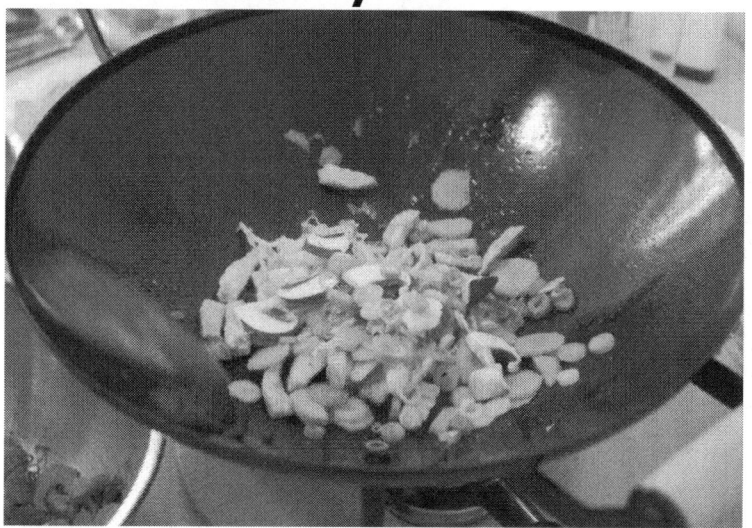

Serving: 2

Prep Time: 10minutes

Cook Time: 20 minutes

Ingredients

- 2 silvered stalks of leeks
- 2 diced up middle sized white onion
- 1 silvered Zucchini
- 2 coarsely diced up tomatoes
- 2 tablespoon of extra virgin olive oil
- 1 tablespoon of grated cheddar
- 1 teaspoon of sea salt
- 1 tablespoon of parsley
- 1 teaspoon of oregano
- ½ a teaspoon of curry powder
- Freshly ground black pepper
- ½ a cup of water

Cooking Directions

1. Take a medium sized pan and add olive oil, heat it up over medium heat
2. Add onions and Saute them until lightly browned
3. Add zucchinis and cook for about 3-4 minutes
4. Pour water and cover up the pan
5. Lower down the heat to low and let it simmer for 10 minutes
6. Add tomatoes and season with some pepper and curry powder
7. Cook for 10 minutes, making sure to keep the lid closed
8. Once done, season with some more parsley and salt
9. Add cheese and serve! Serve with some bread if you require your meal to have greater alkaline value!

Nutrition Values

- Calories: 80
- Fats: 7g
- Carbs: 4g
- Fiber: 1g

Almond And Celery Mix Of Delight! #5

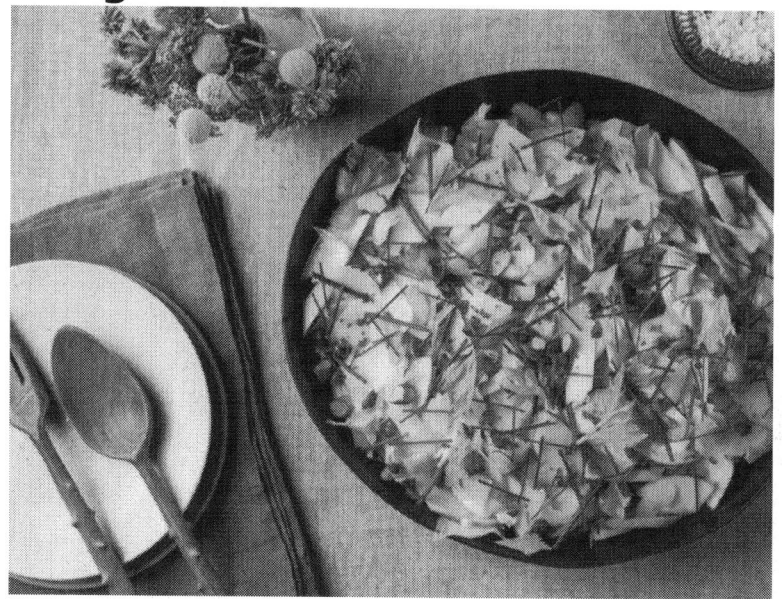

Serving: 2

Prep Time: 60 minutes

Cook Time: 0 minutes

Ingredients

- 10 ounce of sliced up knob celery
- 6-7 ounce of cubed up apples
- 2/3 cups of water
- 1/3 cup of almonds
- ½ of a lemon
- ½ a tablespoon of salt
- Pepper as needed

Cooking Directions

1. Take a medium sized bowl and add apples, celery, and lemon juice
2. Mix everything well
3. Blend your almonds in a blender and add some water to get a very nice and smooth paste
4. Add the paste to a bowl and season with some salt and pepper
5. Mix well and chill for 60 minutes
6. Add the paste to your bowl with apples and serve!

Nutrition Values

- Calories: 221
- Fats: 15g
- Carbs: 23g
- Fiber: 3g

Spicy Tofu Burger (Magical) #6

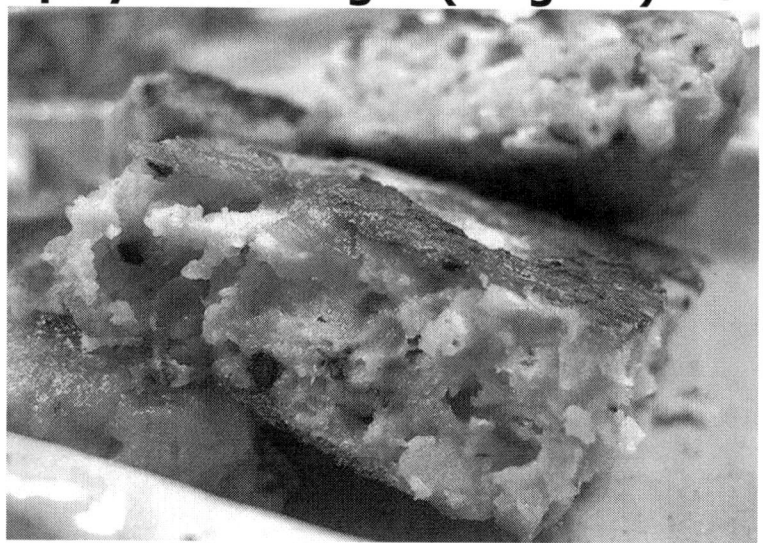

Serving: 4

Prep Time: 5 minutes

Cook Time: 15 minutes

Ingredients

- 500g of firm tofu
- 100g of green bell pepper
- 6 teaspoon of organic chili sauce
- ½ a teaspoon of sea salt
- 2 teaspoon of extra virgin olive oil
- Pepper as needed

Cooking Directions

1. Chop up the tofu, bell peppers and onions into tiny pieces
2. Take a pan and place it over medium heat
3. Add oil and heat it up, add the cut veggies and stir fry for 5 minutes

4. Add tofu and stir fry for another 15 minutes
5. Add chili sauce into the mix and season with some pepper and salt to adjust the flavor accordingly
6. Add water and wet the mixture
7. Serve with alkaline bread, keeping the mixture between two pieces of bread

Nutrition Values

- Calories: 496
- Fats: 13g
- Carbs: 74g
- Fiber: 6g

Special Pasta Ala Pepper and Tomato Sauce #7

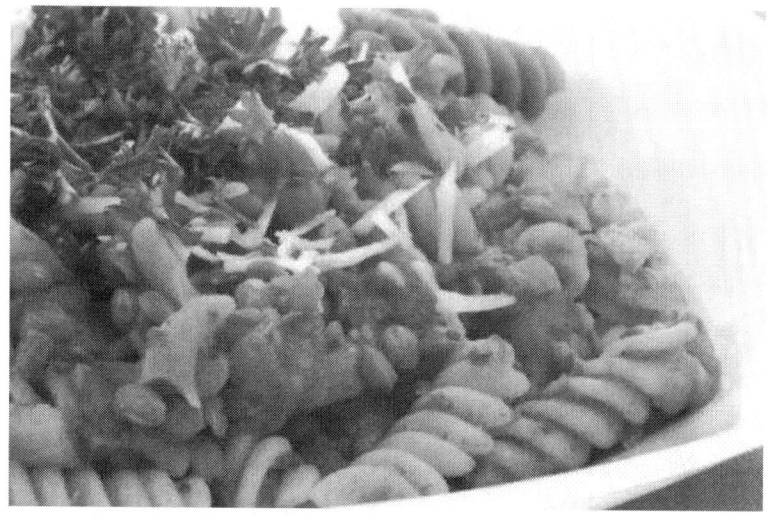

Serving: 4

Prep Time: 5 minutes

Cook Time: 10 minutes

Ingredients

- 500g of vegetable pasta
- 300g of tomatoes
- ½ a cup of sun dried tomatoes
- 1 small sized red bell pepper
- 1 small sized Zucchini
- 1 piece of onion
- 2 pieces of garlic cloves
- 1 piece of chili
- 5 pieces of fresh basil leaves
- 2-3 tablespoon of cold pressed olive oil
- Sea salt as needed
- Pepper as needed

Cooking Directions

1. Cook the pasta properly according to the specified package instructions
2. Cut up the tomatoes, bell pepper, zucchini into fine cubes and chop the chili, garlic, and onions
3. Take a pan and place it over medium heat
4. Add oil and heat up the oil
5. Add onions, chili, pepper, and garlic and fry them for a few minutes
6. Add tomatoes, zucchini and cook for 5-10 minutes more
7. Add basil
8. Season with pepper and salt to adjust the flavor
9. Add pasta on top your serving plate
10. Pour the sauce and season
11. Serve!

Nutrition Values

- Calories: 591
- Fats: 22g
- Carbs: 73g
- Fiber: 5g

Southern Amazing Salad #8

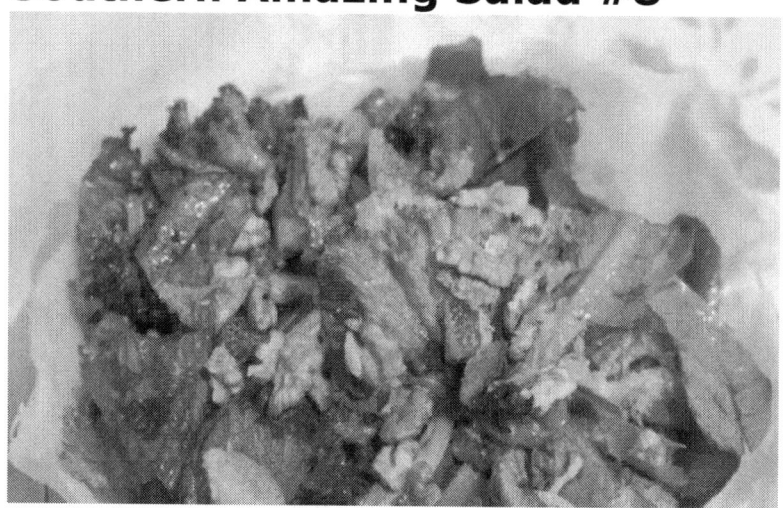

Serving: 2

Prep Time: 15 minutes

Cook Time: 0 minutes

Ingredients

- 5 cups of Romaine lettuce
- ½ a cup of sprouted black beans
- 1 cup of halved cherry tomatoes
- 1 diced avocado
- ¼ cup of chopped almonds
- ½ a cup of fresh cilantro
- ½ a cup of Salsa Fresca

Cooking Directions

1. Take a large sized bowl and add lettuce, tomatoes, beans, almonds, cilantro, avocado, Salsa Fresco
2. Toss everything well and mix them
3. Divide the salad into serving bowls and serve!

Nutrition Values

- Calories: 370
- Fats: 16g
- Carbs: 44g
- Fiber: 14g

A Concoction of Roast Veggies #9

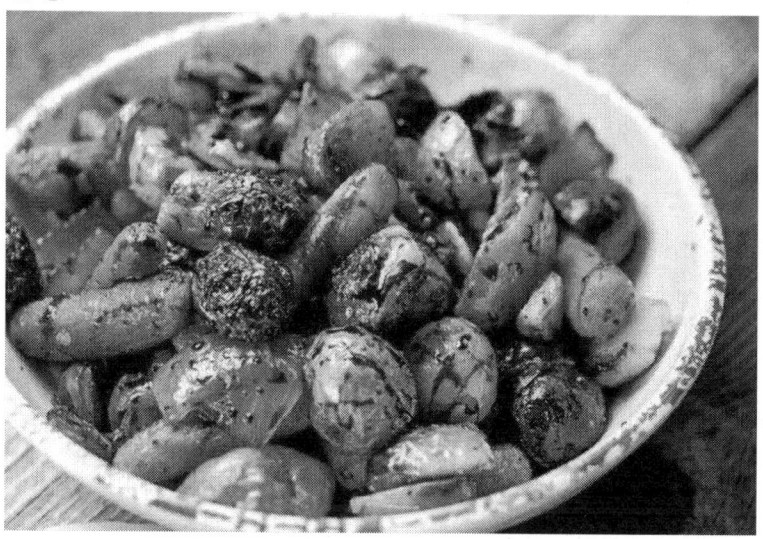

Serving: 2

Prep Time: 10 minutes

Cook Time: 15 minutes

Ingredients

- ½ a bunch of trimmed asparagus
- 1 pint of cherry tomatoes
- ½ a cup of halved mushrooms
- 1 peeled carrots cut up into bite sized portions
- 1 red bell pepper
- 1 yellow bell pepper (both peppers should be deseeded and cut into bite sized portions)
- 1 tablespoon of coconut oil
- 1 tablespoon of garlic powder
- 1 teaspoon of sea salt

Cooking Directions

1. Preheat your oven to a temperature of 425 degrees Fahrenheit
2. Take a bowl and add asparagus, mushrooms, tomatoes, bell pepper and carrot
3. Add coconut milk, salt, garlic powder and toss everything well to ensure that everything mixed
4. Transfer the mixed veggies to a baking pan and place the pan in a pre-heated oven
5. Roast for 15 minutes until they are nice and tender
6. Transfer the roasted veggies to a bowl
7. Divide into serving bowls and enjoy!

Nutrition Values

- Calories: 132
- Fats: 7.3g
- Carbs: 15g
- Fiber: 5g

A Thai Pad Thai #10

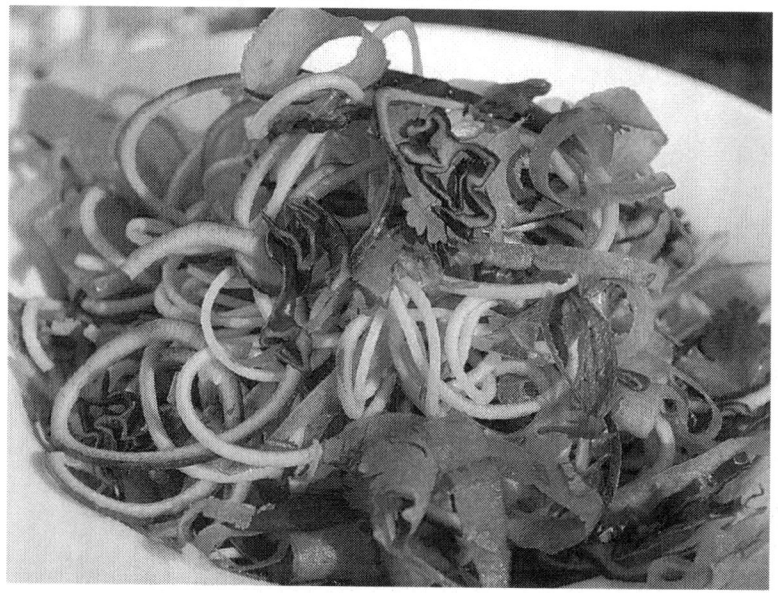

Serving: 2

Prep Time: 10 minutes

Cook Time: 0 minutes

Ingredients

- 4 cups of chopped iceberg lettuce
- 1 cup of bean sprouts
- 2 carrots cut up into thin slices
- 1 piece of zucchini cut up into strips
- 1 finely chopped scallions
- 2 tablespoon of chopped almonds
- 1 lime juice
- 1 clove of garlic
- 1 teaspoon of tamarind paste
- 1 pack of stevia
- ½ a teaspoon of sea salt

Cooking Directions

1. Take a large sized bowl and add lettuce carrots, zucchini, bean sprouts and almonds
2. Take a small sized food processor bowl and add garlic, lime juice, stevia, salt, and blend well
3. Pour the dressing over your veggies and mix well
4. Divide the mixture into serving bowl and enjoy!

Nutrition Values

- Calories: 77
- Fats: 3.2g
- Carbs: 6.4g
- Fiber: 5.5g

Chapter 3: Dinner Recipes

Chinese Cucumber Salad Magnifico #1

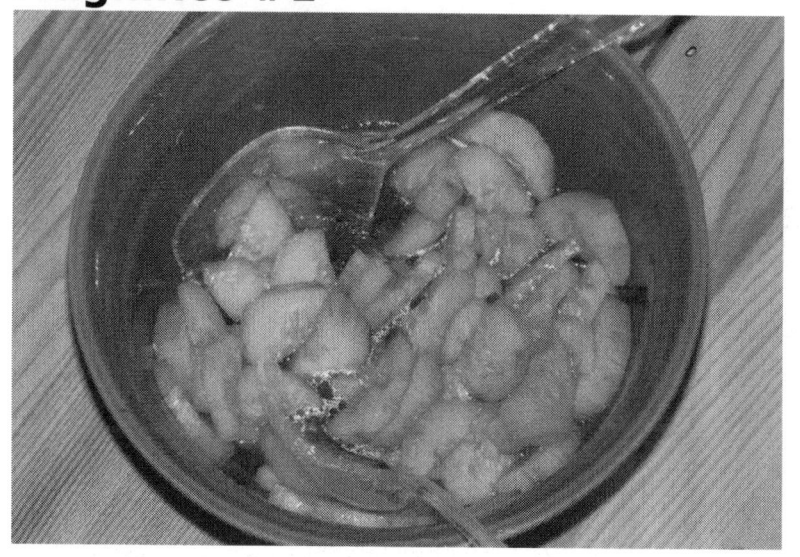

Serving: 4

Prep Time: 15 minutes

Cook Time: 0

Ingredients

- 1 pound of fresh cucumber
- 4 cloves of garlic
- 3 tablespoon of sesame seed oil
- Just a pinch of salt
- Pinch of pepper

Cooking Directions

1. Take a bowl and add oil
2. Add salt and just a pinch of pepper
3. Add minced up garlic to the bowl and toss them well to mix everything up
4. Wash the cucumbers well and cut them in half
5. Cut the halves into slices
6. Add the slices to the bowl and toss them well to ensure that they are coated well
7. Chill the salad in your fridge for 10 minutes
8. Serve!

Nutrition Values

- Calories: 20
- Fats: 0g
- Carbs: 4g
- Fiber: 1g

Mediterranean Alkaline Salad #2

Specialty

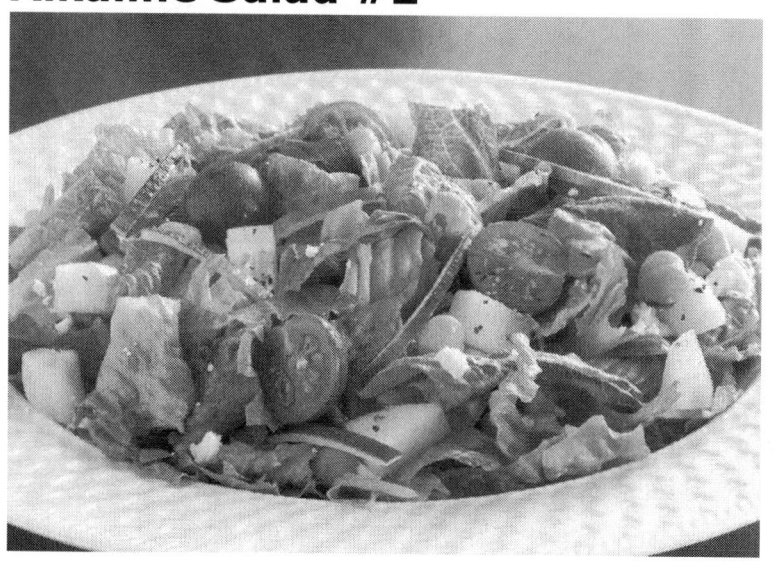

Serving: 3

Prep Time: 10 minutes

Cook Time: 0 minutes

Ingredients

- 1 piece of red bell pepper
- 1 piece of yellow bell pepper
- 3 large pieces of tomatoes
- 10 black olives dipped in oil
- 1 piece of onion
- 1 small sized stalk of leek
- Celery leaves

For Dressing

- 1/3 cup of fresh lemon juice
- ¾ cup of cold pressed olive oil

- 1 teaspoon of garlic powder
- ½ a teaspoon of ground oregano
- ¼ teaspoon of dried rosemary
- 1 teaspoon of dried basil
- ½ teaspoon of ground cumin
- 1 dash of sea salt
- 1 dash of cayenne pepper

Cooking Directions

1. Dice tomatoes and pepper
2. Cut onion, celery leaves, and leeks into strips
3. Take a salad bowl and add the vegetables
4. To prepare the salad, add all of the listed ingredients (salad dressing) to a blender and blitz them well
5. Season with some flax seed
6. Pour the dressing over veggies and toss well to mix up
7. Serve!

Nutrition Values

- Calories: 204
- Fats: 16g
- Carbs: 10g
- Fiber: 1g

Emmenthal Justifiable Soup From Swiss! #3

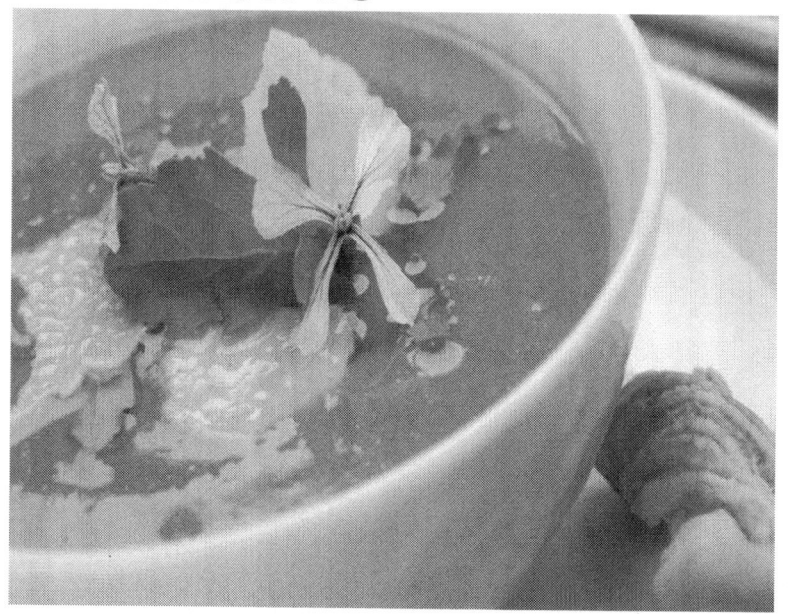

Serving: 2

Prep Time: 5 minutes

Cook Time: 5 minutes

Ingredients

- 2 cups of cauliflower pieces
- 1 cubed up potato
- 2 cups of yeast free vegetable stock
- 3 tablespoon of cubed up Emmenthal cheese
- 2 tablespoon of fresh chives
- 1 tablespoon of pumpkin seeds
- 1 pinch of nutmeg
- 1 pinch of cayenne pepper

Cooking Directions

1. Cook cauliflower and potatoes in vegetable broth to make sure that they are tender
2. Add the tender veggies to a blender and puree them
3. Season the soup with cayenne, nutmeg
4. Season with salt and pepper to adjust the flavor
5. Add Emmenthal cheese, chives and stir well
6. Garnish with pumpkin seeds and serve!

Nutrition Values

- Calories: 351
- Fats: 14g
- Carbs: 28g
- Fiber: 4g

Buckwheat Pasta mixed up with Bell Pepper and Broccoli #4

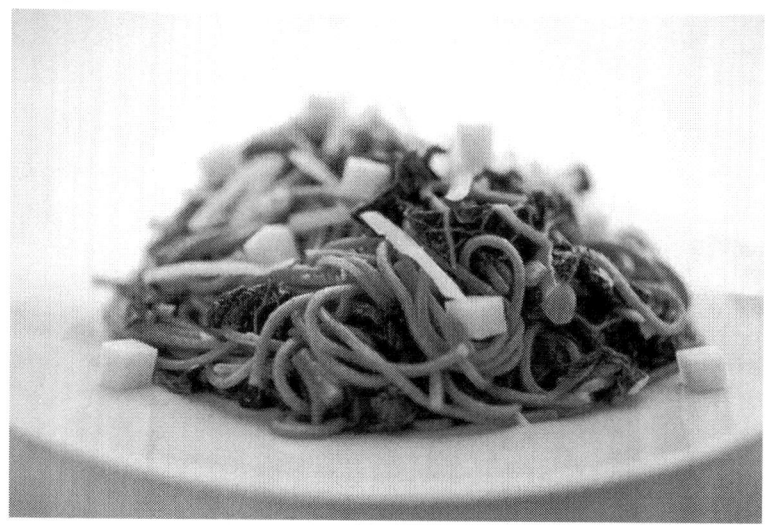

Serving: 3-4

Prep Time: 5 minutes

Cook Time: 10 minutes

Ingredients

- 500g of buckwheat pasta
- 4 tablespoon of extra virgin olive oil cold pressed out
- 2 diced up cloves of garlic
- 1 middle sized white onion ring
- Strips of 1 red bell pepper
- 1 big broccoli head cut up into florets
- 3 diced up middle sized tomatoes
- 3 sliced up carrots
- 1 tablespoon of fresh lemon juice

- 1 teaspoon of oregano
- 1 teaspoon of yeast free vegetable broth
- Sea salt as needed
- Pepper as needed

Cooking Directions

1. the vegetables into bite sized portions
2. Take a pot of water and add salt
3. Heat it up and buckwheat pasta. Cook it to Al Dente
4. Take another pot and add broccoli and water. Cook these as well
5. Take a pan and place it over medium heat
6. Add 2 tablespoon of olive oil and add onions and garlic
7. Saute them
8. Take out and keep it on the side
9. Add 2 tablespoon of oil to the pan and cook veggies until tender
10. Make sure to first cook the carrots, then bell pepper and finally tomatoes
11. Drain the cooked broccoli and add the broccoli and onions to the pan with vegetables
12. Add lemon juice, oregano, and vegetable broth
13. Season with salt and pepper to adjust the flavor
14. Stir well
15. Add the veggie mix over your buckwheat pasta and serve!

Nutrition Values

- Calories: 583
- Fats: 26g
- Carbs:61g
- Fiber: 4g

Artichoke Sauce Ala Quinoa Pasta! #5

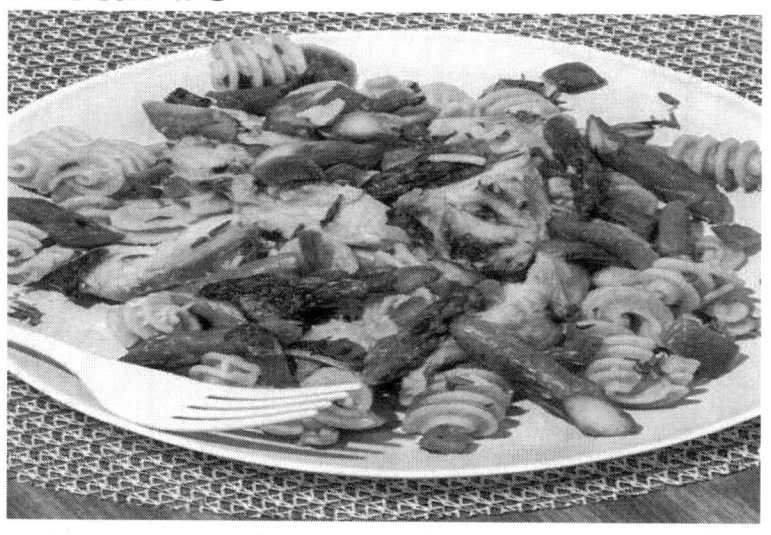

Serving: 4

Prep Time: 15 minutes

Cook Time: 0

<u>Ingredients</u>

- 7 ounce or 200g spelled pasta
- 8 ounce or 220g of frozen artichoke
- 5 ounce of fresh tomatoes
- 1 medium sized onion
- 1 clove of garlic
- 1 ounce of pine nuts
- 1 teaspoon of yeast free vegetable stock
- 3 tablespoon of fresh basil
- ½ a teaspoon of yeast free vegetable stock
- 3 tablespoon of fresh basil
- ½ a teaspoon of organic sea salt
- 1 pinch of cayenne pepper

- 2 tablespoon of cold pressed extra virgin olive oil

Cooking Directions

1. Prepare your Artichokes by cooking them gently until they show a tender texture
2. Cook the pasta to Al Dente following the instructions on your packet
3. Take out your tomatoes and cut them up into cubes
4. Chop up the onions, garlic, and basil into bite sized portions
5. Take a pan and add 2 tablespoons of olive oil over medium heat
6. Add pine nuts, garlic, and onion and stir them for a few minutes
7. Take another bowl and add ½ a cup of water and dissolve yeast free veggie stock
8. Add the mixture to the pan
9. Simmer it over low heat and keep stirring it for 2 minutes
10. Once done, add basil and season with cayenne pepper and salt
11. Pour the sauce over your pasta
12. Serve!

Nutrition Values

- Calories: 286
- Fats: 13g
- Carbs: 26g
- Fiber: 3g

The Mighty Indian Curry Of Lentil #6

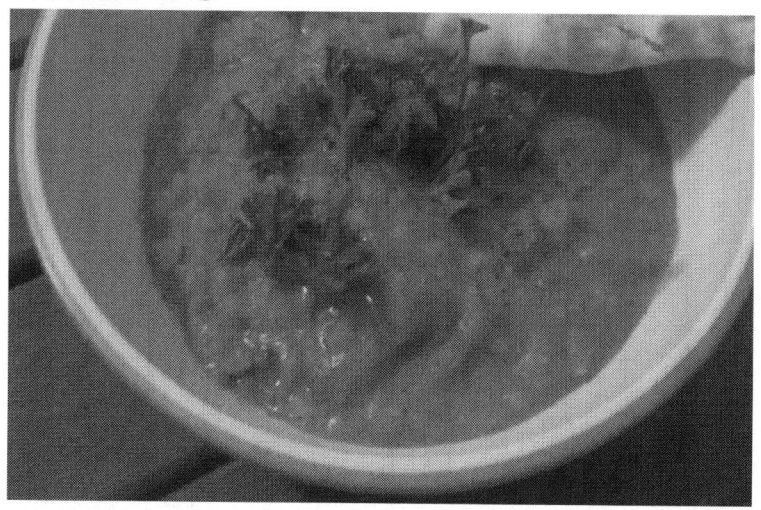

Serving: 4-6

Prep Time: 10 minutes

Cook Time: 10

Ingredients

- 1 cup of fine red lentils
- 2 pieces of green chilies
- ½ a teaspoon of cumin seeds
- ½ a teaspoon of turmeric
- 1 inch piece of grated ginger
- 1 minced up clove of garlic
- 1 sliced of medium onion
- 2 medium sized tomatoes
- 1 tablespoon of oil
- Salt as needed
- Chopped up cilantro for garnish
- Lime juice is you desire

Cooking Directions

1. Take a bowl and add water
2. Add lentils and soak them in water for about 6 hours
3. Take a pan and place it over low heat
4. Pour water alongside the lentils and let the mixture boil
5. Add a pinch of turmeric
6. Simmer until it reaches your desired level of consistency
7. Take it out and add them to another bowl
8. Take another pan and heat up oil over medium heat
9. Add onions, ginger, cumin, and turmeric
10. Add tomatoes, chilies and cook the mixture with some salt as well until they are nice
11. Add the lentils to this mixture and bring it to a boil
12. Once boiling point is reached take it off the stove immediately and squeeze a bit of lemon on top
13. Garnish with cilantro and serve over rice

Nutrition Values

- Calories: 421
- Fats: 6g
- Carbs: 79g
- Fiber: 59g

Savory Deluxe Mix Of Veggies #7

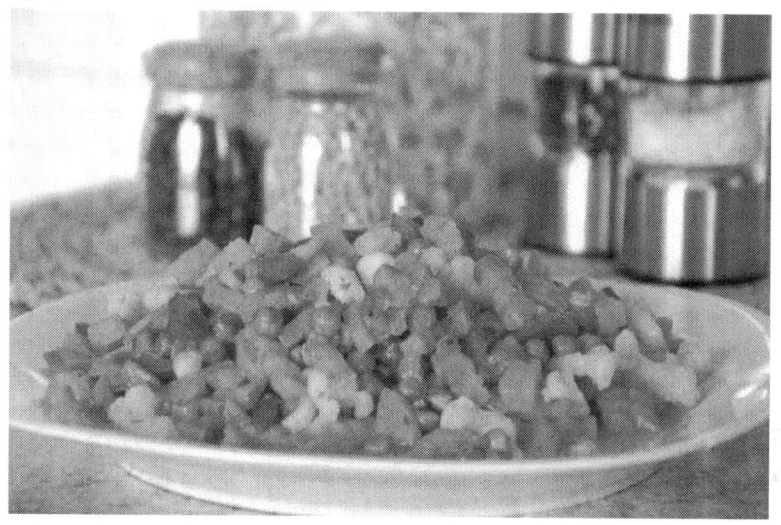

Serving: 4-6

Prep Time: 10 minutes

Cook Time: 10

Ingredients

- 2 tablespoon of vegetable oil
- 1 chopped up large sized onion
- 1 seed and chopped up poblano chili
- 1 piece of seeded and chopped up red bell pepper
- 3 cloves of minced up garlic
- 1 and a ½ teaspoon of chili powder
- 1 and a ½ teaspoon of cumin powder
- 2 cups of cooked bean all rinsed up and drained
- 2 and a ½ cup of vegetable stock
- 3 teaspoon of lime juice

- 4 tablespoon of chopped up cilantro

Cooking Directions

1. Take a medium sized pot and place it over medium heat
2. Add oil and allow it to heat up
3. Add onions and Saute them for a while
4. Add red bell pepper, jalapeno, poblano chili, garlic and cook for about 2-3 minutes until the veggies are finely cooked
5. Add spices and give them a stir
6. Add beans with the vegetable stock
7. Bring the whole mixture to a boil and lower down the temperature to low
8. Cook for 15 minutes
9. Stir in lemon juice and garnish with cilantro
10. Serve!

Pro Tip: The dish can be made more lucrative with the addition of mushrooms, cabbage, potatoes, etc.

Keep in mind not to add any dairy or sugar products as they will alter the alkalinity of the meal.

Nutrition Values

- Calories: 485
- Fats: 13g
- Carbs: 71g
- Fiber: 12g

Very Wild Avocado Salad #8

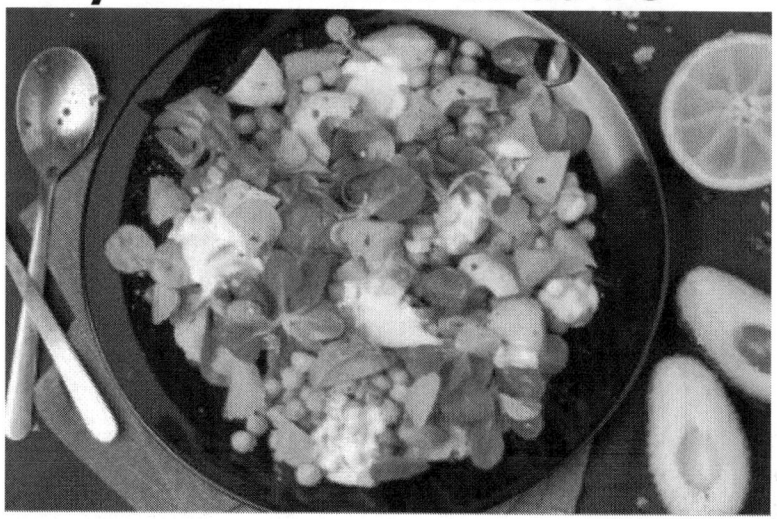

Serving: 2

Prep Time: 10 minutes

Cook Time: 0 minutes

Ingredients

- 1 piece of avocado
- 1 bunch of wild garlic
- 3 pieces of tomatoes
- 1 piece of red bell pepper
- 2 tablespoon of cold pressed extra virgin olive oil
- Sea salt as needed
- 1 pinch of cayenne

Cooking Directions

1. Cut up your peeled up avocados
2. Cut up bell peppers into half, and cut up the half into thin slices

3. Chop up the tomatoes into small sized cubes and add them to a medium bowl
4. Chop up the wild garlic into small pieces and add them to a bowl
5. Pour olive oil and toss everything well
6. Add pepper and salt to season it
7. Serve!

Nutrition Values

- Calories: 213
- Fats: 21g
- Carbs: 2g
- Fiber: 5g

The Mysterious Alkaline Veggies and Rice (Wilde) #9

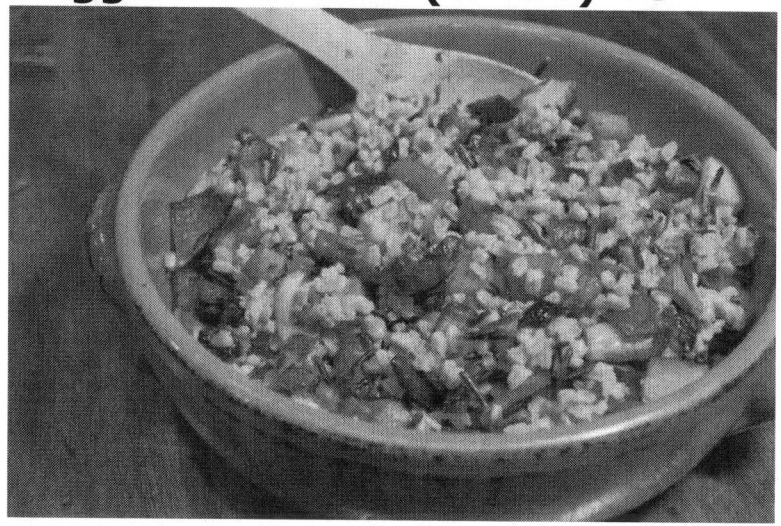

Serving: 4

Prep Time: 10 minutes

Cook Time: 5 minutes

Ingredients

- 1 cup of wild rice
- 1 cup of Pak Choi
- 1 cup o Broccoli
- 1 cup of Young Beans
- 2 cups of Carrots
- 1 cup of bean sprout
- ½ a cup of vegetable broth
- 1 piece of chili
- 1 fresh juice of lime
- Cilantro as needed
- Basil as required
- Seas Salt as required

Cooking Directions

1. Chop up the Pak Choi, carrots, beans, bean sprouts, and broccoli
2. Add them to a pan and pour vegetable broth
3. Steam fry the mixture until they are fully cooked and are a bit crunchy
4. Take a mortar and pestle and add cilantro and chopped up chili
5. Pour lime juice and mix well to prepare the dressing
6. Take a serving platter add rice, add the prepped vegetables
7. Serve by pouring the dressing over them!

Nutrition Values

- Calories: 200
- Fats: 2g
- Carbs: 33g
- Fiber: 2g

Beautifully Curried Eggplant #10

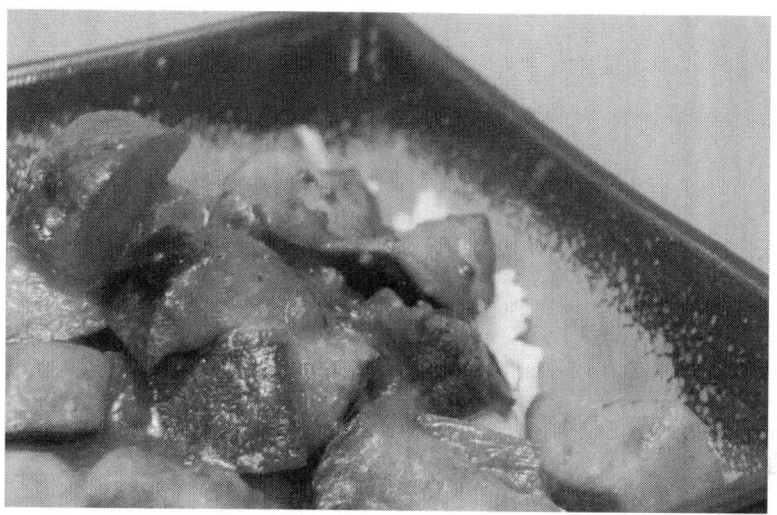

Serving: 2

Prep Time: 5 minutes

Cook Time: 5 minutes

Ingredients

- 1 piece of roasted eggplant (make sure to remove the contents from the shell and reserve juice from about 1 lemon)
- 1 teaspoon of sea salt
- 1 teaspoon of curry powder
- Water as required
- Cooked quinoa required for serving

Cooking Directions

1. Take a food processor and add eggplant, lemon juice, sesame oil, salt, curry powder and blend the whole mixture well

2. Take a small sized saucepan and place it over medium heat
3. Add the eggplant mix to your saucepan and gently warm it for about 5 minutes
4. Add water to thin it if required
5. Serve the curried eggplants over some delicious quinoa!

Nutrition Values

- Calories: 81
- Fats: 2.8g
- Carbs: 14g
- Fiber: 8g

Chapter 4: Dessert Recipes

Magnificent Coconut Ice Cream Sundae #1

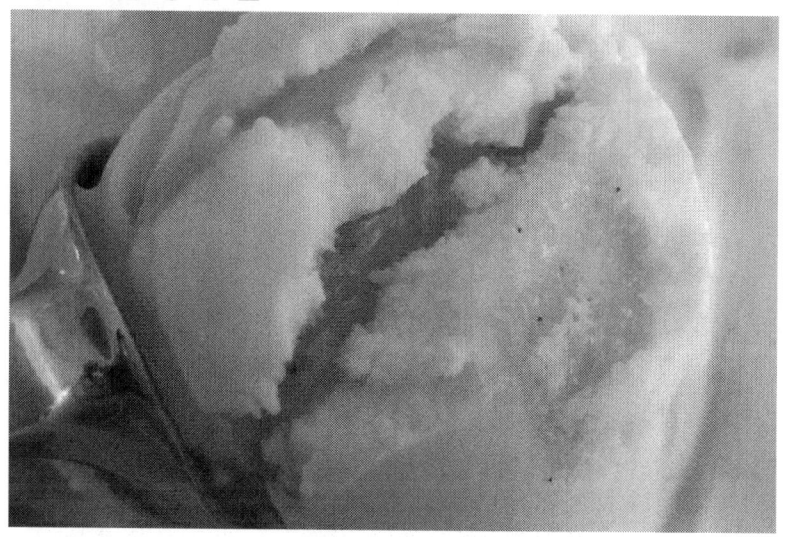

Serving: 4

Prep Time: 5 minutes

Freeze Time: overnight

Ingredients

- 2 cans of full fat unsweetened coconut milk
- 1 cup of coconut sugar
- 1/8 teaspoon of sea salt
- 1 vanilla bean split lengthwise and seeds scraped out
- Topping such as bananas, unsweetened coconut, chopped almonds and strawberries

Cooking Directions

1. Prepare your blender and add coconut milk, salt, coconut sugar, vanilla bean seeds mix everything well
2. Transfer the mixture to a freezer-safe bowl and let it freeze overnight
3. Add about 2 scoops of your prepared ice cream to a small sized bowl and garnish with your assorted selection of alkaline friendly toppings

Nutrition Values

- Calories: 306
- Fats: 22g
- Carbs: 30g
- Fiber: 2.6g

All Purpose Thanksgiving Pudding #2

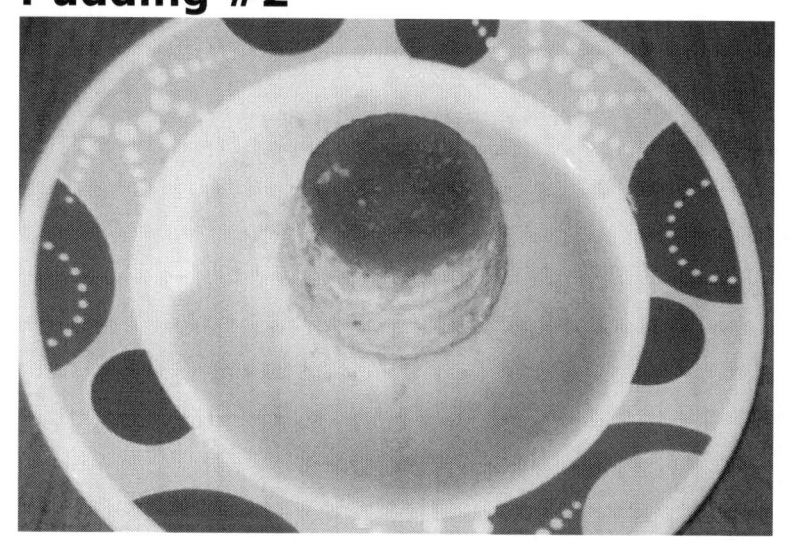

Serving: 8

Prep Time: 10 minutes

Cook Time: 60 minutes

Ingredients

- 1 can of unsweetened pumpkin puree
- ½ a cup of unsweetened coconut milk
- 1 teaspoon of cinnamon
- ¼ teaspoon of sea salt
- ½ a cup of raisins
- ½ a cup of peeled, diced and cored apples
- Coconut whipped cream (optional)

Cooking Directions

1. Preheat your oven to a temperature of 350 degrees Fahrenheit

2. Take a food processor and add pumpkin, cinnamon, coconut milk, salt and nutmeg and mix them until they are aerated
3. Add raisins and the apples
4. Pulse to combine
5. Take a 9 inch baking dish and add the mixture
6. Bake for about 60 minutes until the top it slightly cracked
7. Serve with some coconut whipped cream (optional)

Nutrition Values

- Calories: 69
- Fats: 0.6g
- Carbs: 16g
- Fiber:2.2g

Dates For A Valentine's Day Date #3

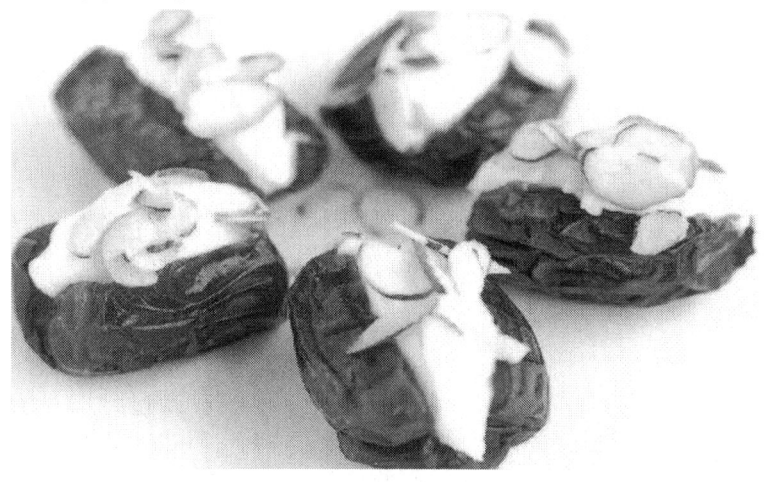

Serving: 1

Prep Time: 10 minutes

Cook Time: 0 minutes

Ingredients

- 4 pitted Mejdool dates
- 4 halved almonds
- ¼ cup of shredded unsweetened coconut

Cooking Directions

1. Take a sharp knife and slice up the dates lengthwise
2. Make sure to cut them all the way through
3. Press the open dates and lay them on a flat surface
4. Take a rolling pin and flatten the dates
5. Place one piece of almond on the flattened date and fold the other side over

6. Enclose the almond between the date halves
7. Repeat until all the dates are used
8. Press each of the dates into your coconut
9. Have fun eating!

Nutrition Values

- Calories: 178
- Fats: 8g
- Carbs: 27g
- Fiber: 4.3g

Crispy Fruit Mix #4

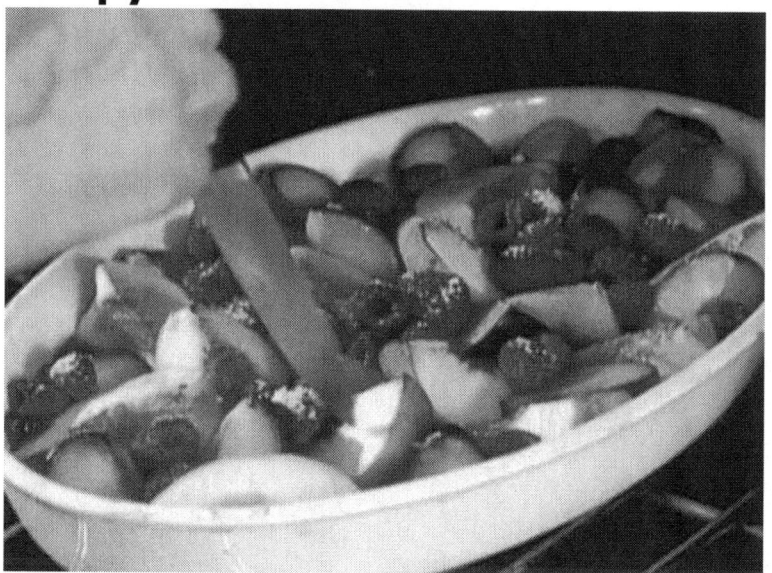

Serving: 6

Prep Time: 15 minutes

Cook Time: 15 minutes

Ingredients

- Cooking spray for grease
- 2 cups of chopped summer fruits, plums, and strawberries
- 1 pack of stevia
- 1 vanilla bean split lengthwise and seeds scraped out
- 1 and a ½ cups of raw almonds
- ½ a cup of raw almonds
- ½ a cup of unsweetened coconut shredded
- 1 tablespoon of melted oil
- ¼ teaspoon of sea salt

Cooking Directions

1. Preheat your oven to a temperature of 350 degrees Fahrenheit
2. Take a 9 inch baking dish and grease it up with cooking spray
3. Take a large sized saucepan and place it over medium heat
4. Add chopped up fruits, vanilla bean, and stevia
5. Stir well and bring the mix to a boil
6. Take a food processor and add almonds, salt, coconut oil, and pulse the mixture until a crumbly mix forms
7. Transfer the fruits to your baking dish
8. Top it up with the almond coconut mix
9. Bake for 15 minutes
10. Serve!

Nutrition Values

- Calories: 240
- Fats: 16g
- Carbs: 20g
- Fiber: 5.8g

Slightly Crispy Rice Treatlets #5

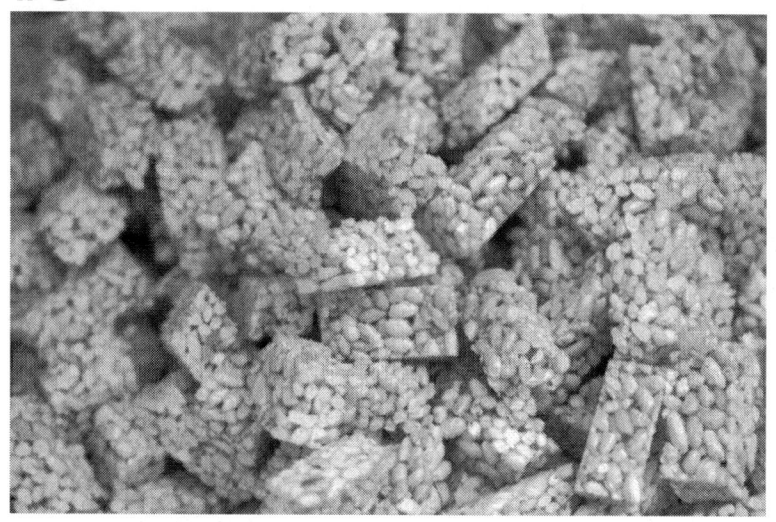

Serving: 12

Prep Time: 5 minutes

Cook Time: 1 minute

Ingredients

- Cooking spray for grease
- 2/3 cup of brown rice syrup
- ¼ cup of coconut oil
- 1 vanilla bean split lengthwise and seeds scraped out
- ¼ teaspoon of sea salt
- 4 cups of brown rice crisp

Cooking Directions

1. Take an 9 inch baking pan and grease it up with cooking spray

2. Take a medium sized saucepan and place it over medium heat
3. Add brown rice syrup, coconut oil and bring the mix to a boil for about 1 minute
4. Add vanilla bean seeds alongside salt
5. Take a large sized bowl and add rice cereal
6. Pour the syrup mixture over your cereal and mix well
7. Transfer the mixture to your pan
8. Spray your hands using cooking spray and use your hands press the rice mix and distribute it evenly
9. Let it chill for 45 minutes
10. Once done, cut it up into 12 bars and serve!

Nutrition Values

- Calories: 104
- Fats: 4.6g
- Carbs: 15g
- Fiber: 4.6g

Mystical Indian Aloo Gobi #6

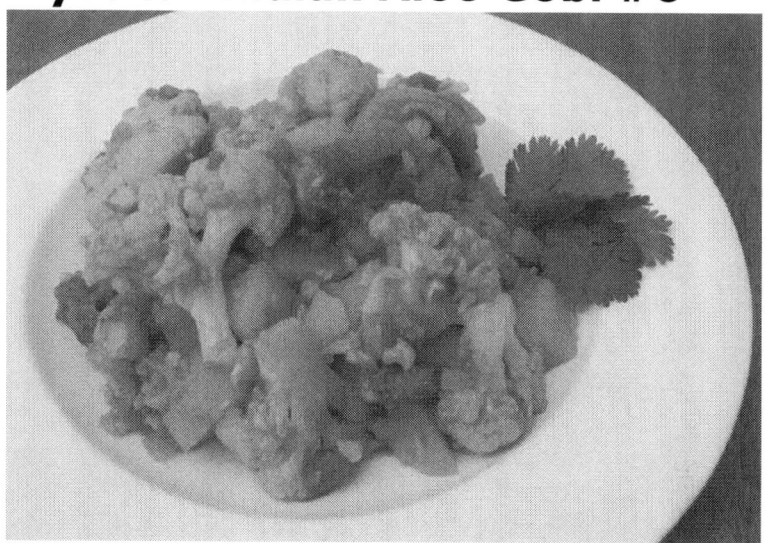

Serving: 2

Prep Time: 5 minutes

Cook Time: 10 minutes

<u>Ingredients</u>

- 20g of fresh ginger
- 2 cloves of fresh garlic
- 4 pieces of green chilies
- 2 large sized onions
- 400g of diced up tomatoes
- 750g of cauliflower
- 2 teaspoon of Turmeric
- 2 teaspoon of Garam masala
- 125ml of cold pressed extra virgin olive oil
- 1/3 cup of coriander and cilantro leaves
- Salt as need
- 1/3 cup of mint
- 2 teaspoon of cayenne pepper

- 3 cups of water

Cooking Directions

1. Take a grinder and grind your garlic, chili, and ginger
2. Take a pan and place it over medium heat
3. Add oil and heat it up for about 3 minutes
4. Add onions and Saute until they are golden
5. Add the grinded paste and stir well for a few seconds
6. Add tomatoes, salt, turmeric, Garam Masala, chili and cook for about 5 minutes until the tomatoes are pulpy
7. Add the remaining ingredients and stir for 3 minutes
8. Add water and cook until the vegetables are done and thick sauce forms
9. Serve the mixture over Basmati Rice

Nutrition Values

- Calories: 178
- Fats: 5g
- Carbs: 25g
- Fiber: 5g

Crazy Soy Pudding #7

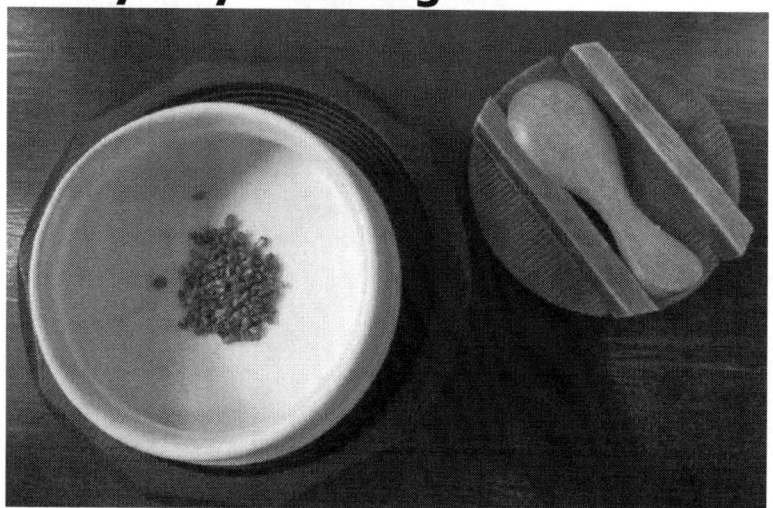

Serving: 4

Prep Time: 10 minutes

Cook Time: 0 minutes

Ingredients

- 1 cup of fresh almond milk (prepare from the previous recipe)
- 2 avocados
- Lime of 1 juice
- 2 scoops of Soy Powder
- 1 package of Stevia
- 6-8 pieces of ice cubes

Cooking Directions

1. Open up your blender and add all of the ingredients
2. Mix them at full speed until a smooth pudding like mixture forms

3. Pour the pudding into a bowl and let it chill
4. Serve!

Nutrition Values

- Calories: 324
- Fats: 3g
- Carbs: 64g
- Fiber: 5g

Mouthwatering Banana Muffins #8

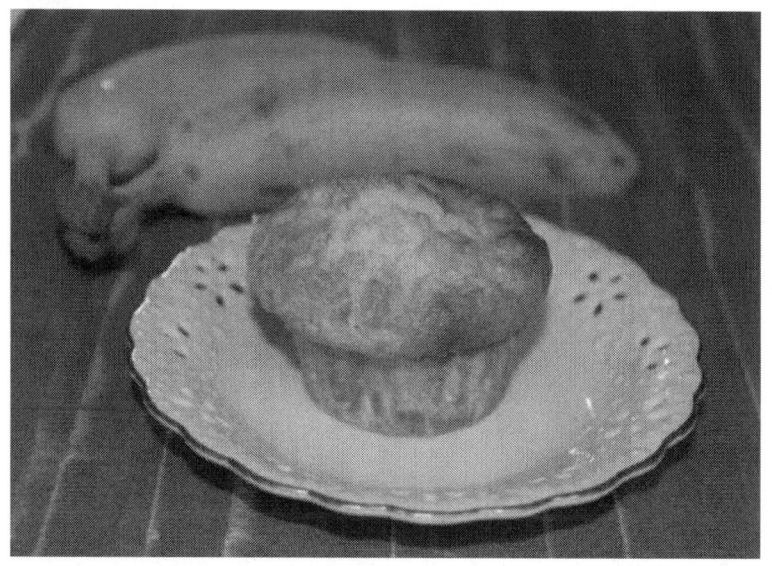

Serving: 12

Prep Time: 5 minutes

Cook Time: 18 minutes

Ingredients

- Cooking spray as grease
- 2 pieces of ripe bananas
- 1 cup of dates
- ½ a cup of roasted creamy almond butter
- ½ a cup of coconut flour
- ¼ cup of melted coconut oil
- 2 teaspoon of baking soda
- ½ a teaspoon of sea salt
- 1 vanilla bean split lengthwise with seeds scraped out

Cooking Directions

1. Preheat your oven to a temperature of 350 degrees Fahrenheit
2. Prepare your muffin pan by lining them up with liners
3. Grease the liners with cooking spray
4. Take a food processor and add bananas, dates and blend well
5. Add almond butter, coconut oil, coconut flour, salt and baking soda alongside vanilla bean seeds
6. Process well until beautiful batter forms
7. Fill up the muffin tins with the batter, making sure to fill each of them to about 2/3rd full
8. Bake for 18 minutes, making sure to check the center using a toothpick to ensure that it comes out clean (if it does, then it's fully cooked)
9. Let it cool and serve!

Nutrition Values

- Calories: 181
- Fats: 10g
- Carbs: 21g
- Fiber: 2.6g

Mr. Clause's Stuffed Avocado #9

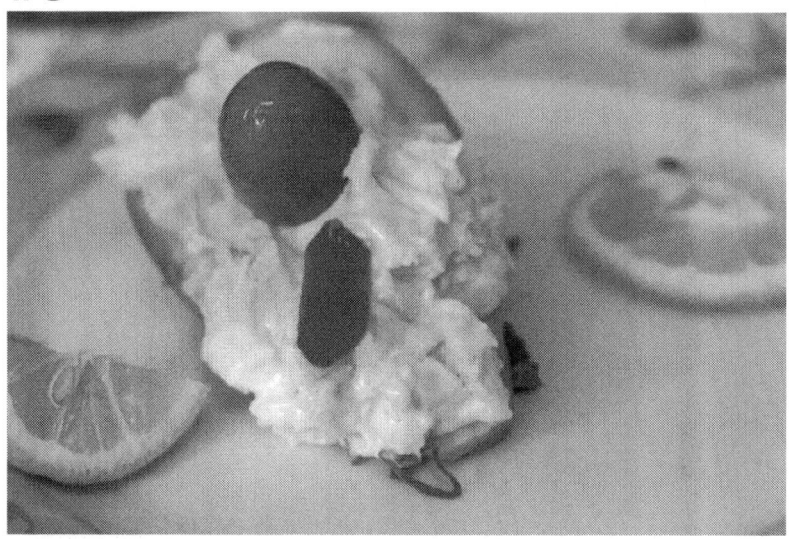

Serving: 2

Prep Time: 15 minutes

Cook Time: 0 minutes

Ingredients

- 1 piece of fully ripe Avocado
- ½ of a tomato
- 1 teaspoon of minced onion
- 1 tablespoon of fresh basil
- 1 teaspoon of fresh oregano
- 1 tablespoon of fresh lime juice
- 4 tablespoon of cold pressed extra virgin olive oil
- Sea salt as needed
- Pepper as needed

Cooking Directions

1. Add your ripped avocado to a cutting board and cut it up in half and deseed it
2. Season the halves with pepper and salt
3. Take a bowl and add chopped tomatoes and minced onions
4. Pour lemon juice and olive oil to the tomato mixture and mix well
5. Scoop up the mixture to the avocado pit holes
6. Sprinkle a bit of basil leaves and oregano
7. Serve and enjoy!

Nutrition Values

- Calories: 324
- Fats: 44
- Carbs: 66g
- Fiber: 15g

Gorgeous Garlic Cabbage #10

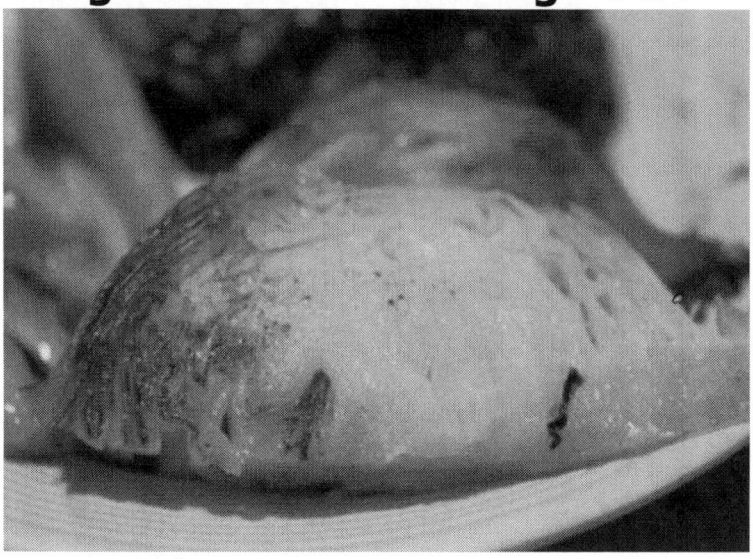

Serving: 4

Prep Time: 5 minutes

Cook Time: 45 minutes

Ingredients

- 1 piece of fully ripe Avocado
- ½ of a tomato
- 1 teaspoon of minced onion
- 1 tablespoon of fresh basil
- 1 teaspoon of fresh oregano
- 1 tablespoon of fresh lime juice
- 4 tablespoon of cold pressed extra virgin olive oil
- Sea salt as needed
- Pepper as needed

Cooking Directions

1. Preheat your oven to a temperature of 425 degrees Fahrenheit
2. Add the cabbage slices to a baking pan and brush both sides of the slice with coconut oil
3. Rub the slices with garlic and sprinkle a bit of salt
4. Transfer the pan to your oven and roast for 20 minutes
5. Flip over and roast for another 20-25 minutes
6. Serve!

Nutrition Values

- Calories: 90
- Fats: 5.3g
- Carbs: 10g
- Fiber: 4.5g

Chapter 5: Fantastic Smoothie Recipes

A Pina Colada For The Adventurers #1

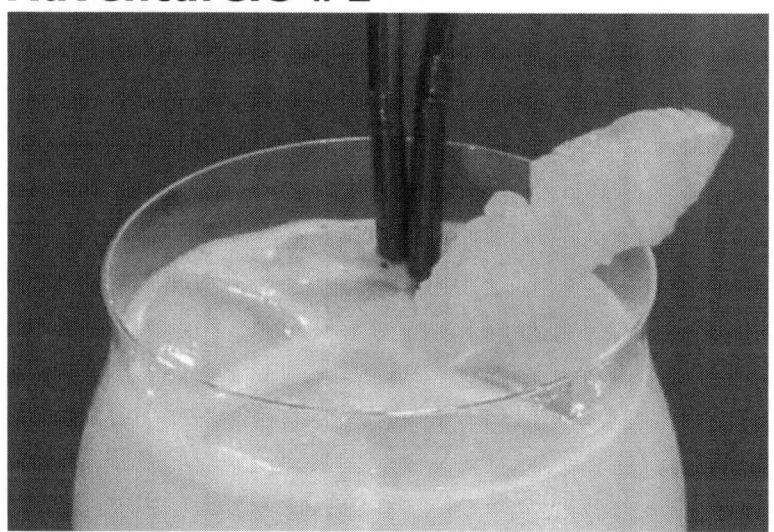

Serving: 1

Prep Time: 2 minutes

Cook Time: 0 minutes

Ingredients

- ½ a cup of unsweetened coconut milk
- 2 and a ½ cups of fresh pineapple chunks
- 1 cup of ice cubes

Cooking Directions

1. Prepare your blender and add coconut milk, ice, and pineapple

2. Blend the mixture until smooth
3. Serve chilled!

Nutrition Values

- Calories: 175
- Fats: 3.2g
- Carbs: 38g
- Fiber: 3.8g

Mango and Papaya Raspberry Smoothie #2

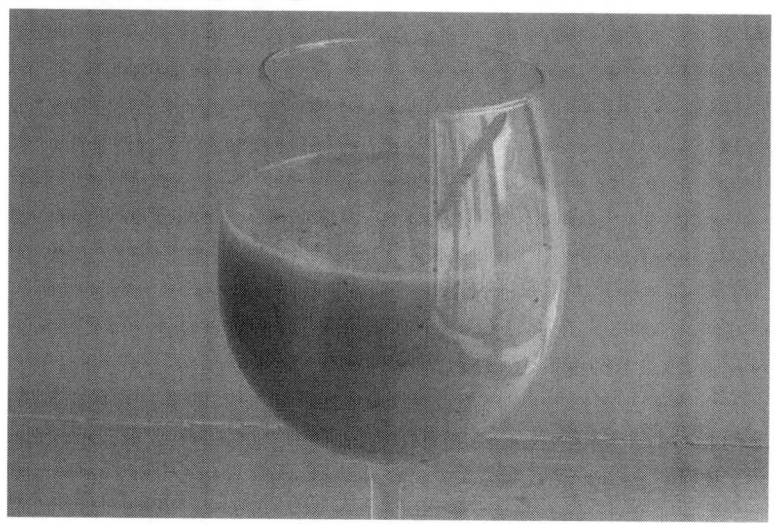

Serving: 1

Prep Time: 2 minutes

Cook Time: 0 minutes

Ingredients

- ¼ cup of raspberries
- ¾ cup of frozen mango pieces
- ½ of a medium sized papaya, chopped up and seeds removed

Cooking Directions

1. Prepare your blender and add mango, raspberries, and papaya
2. Blend the mixture until smooth
3. Serve chilled!

Nutrition Values

- Calories: 153
- Fats: 0.6g
- Carbs: 39g
- Fiber: 6.7g

Sensuous Banana Nut Bread Smoothie #3

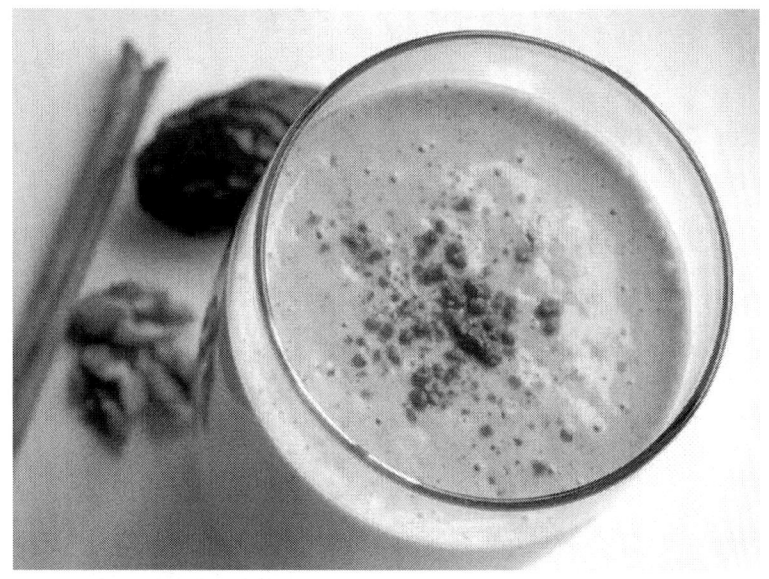

Serving: 1

Prep Time: 2 minutes

Cook Time: 0 minutes

Ingredients

- 1 cup of filtered water
- 1 peeled and medium banana
- 1/4 cup of raw almonds
- ½ a teaspoon of cinnamon
- ¼ teaspoon of nutmeg
- 1 whole vanilla bean split lengthwise with seeds scraped out
- ½ a cup of ice cubes

Cooking Directions

1. Prepare your blender and add water, almonds, banana, nutmeg, cinnamon, vanilla bean seeds and ice
2. Blend the mixture until smooth
3. Serve chilled!

Nutrition Values

- Calories: 254
- Fats: 12g
- Carbs: 33g
- Fiber: 7.2g

Honorable Orange Potion of Health #4

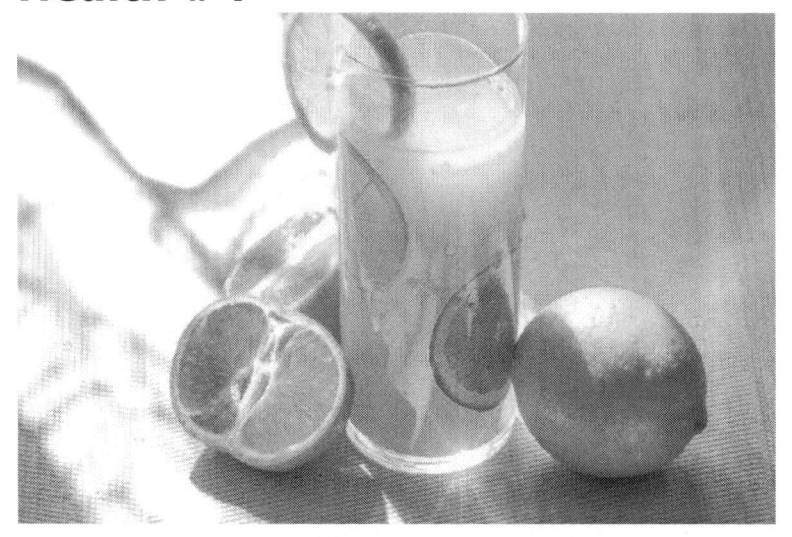

Serving: 1

Prep Time: 2 minutes

Cook Time: 0 minutes

Ingredients

- 6 ounce of freshly squeezed orange juice
- 1 ounce of unsweetened coconut milk
- 1 medium sized frozen banana cut up into chunks
- 1 vanilla bean split lengthwise and seeds scraped out
- 1 pack of stevia

Cooking Directions

1. Prepare your blender and add orange juice, banana, coconut milk, vanilla bean seeds and stevia

2. Blend the mixture until smooth
3. Serve chilled!

Nutrition Values

- Calories: 184
- Fats: 0.3g
- Carbs: 44g
- Fiber: 3.8g

Cherry and Chocolate Mixture #5

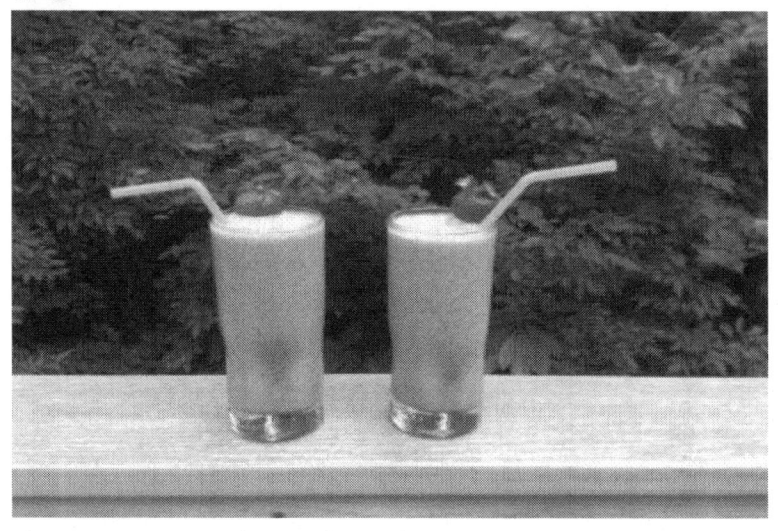

Serving: 1

Prep Time: 2 minutes

Cook Time: 0 minutes

Ingredients

- ½ a cup of frozen dark cherries
- ¾ cup of filtered water
- 1 teaspoon of Dutch-processed cocoa powder
- 1 pack of stevia

Cooking Directions

1. Prepare your blender and add water, cocoa powder, cherries, stevia
2. Blend the mixture until smooth
3. Serve chilled!

Nutrition Values
- Calories: 60
- Fats: 0.6g
- Carbs: 13g
- Fiber: 0.5g

Conclusion

I would like to take a moment here and thank you again for purchasing and downloading my book.

I really do hope that you enjoyed reading the book as much as I enjoyed writing it.

The main aim of this book was to not only introduce you to the world of Alkaline Diet but also give you the opportunity to try out the recipes for yourself and see the changes first hand.

Keep in mind that this is only the tip of the Ice Berg and there's much more to learn about Alkaline Diet.

I bit you farewell.

Stay blessed and Stay Healthy!

God Bless!

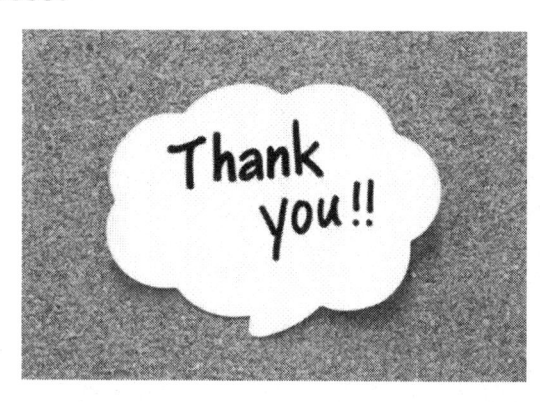

© **Copyright 2017 – Sheldon Miller - All rights reserved.**

In no way is it legal to reproduce, duplicate, or transmit any part of this document by either electronic means or in printed format. Recording of this publication is strictly prohibited, and any storage of this material is not allowed unless with written permission from the publisher. All rights reserved.

The information provided herein is stated to be truthful and consistent, in that any liability, regarding inattention or otherwise, by any usage or abuse of any policies, processes, or directions contained within is the solitary and complete responsibility of the recipient reader. Under no circumstances will any legal liability or blame be held against the publisher for any reparation, damages, or monetary loss due to the information herein, either directly or indirectly.
Respective authors own all copyrights not held by the publisher.

Legal Notice:
This book is copyright protected. This is only for personal use. You cannot amend, distribute, sell, use, quote or paraphrase any part or the content within this book without the consent of the author or copyright owner. Legal action will be pursued if this is breached.

Disclaimer Notice:
Please note the information contained within this document is for educational and entertainment purposes only. Every attempt has been made to

provide accurate, up to date and reliable, complete information. No warranties of any kind are expressed or implied. Readers acknowledge that the author is not engaging in the rendering of legal, financial, medical or professional advice.

By reading this document, the reader agrees that under no circumstances are we responsible for any losses, direct or indirect, which are incurred as a result of the use of information contained within this document, including, but not limited to, — errors, omissions, or inaccuracies.

Made in the USA
Lexington, KY
15 March 2018